HEALTH COUNTS

A Fat and Calorie Guide

Kaiser Permanente

John Wiley & Sons, Inc.

New York • Chichester • Brisbane • Toronto • Singapore

Publisher: Therese A. Zak
Editor: Claire Thompson
Managing Editor: Kate Bradford
Design and Production: Rob Mauhar and Bill Stachura, The Coriolis Group

In recognition of the importance of preserving what has been written, it is a policy of John Wiley & Sons, Inc. to have books of enduring value published in the United States printed on acid-free paper, and we exert our best efforts to that end.

This publication is designed to provide accurate and authoritative information in regard to the subject matter covered. It is sold with the understanding that the publisher is not engaged in rendering legal, accounting, or other professional service. If legal advice or other expert assistance is required, the services of a competent professional person should be sought. FROM A DECLARATION OF PRINCIPLES JOINTLY ADOPTED BY A COMMITTEE OF THE AMERICAN BAR ASSOCIATION AND A COMMITTEE OF PUBLISHERS.

Library of Congress Cataloging-in-Publication Data

Health counts: a fat and calorie guide / Kaiser Permanente.
       p. cm.
     Includes bibliographical references.
     ISBN 0-471-52949-4
     1. Low-fat diet. 2. Low-calorie diet. I. Kaiser Permanente.
RM237.75.H43   1990
613.2'5--dc20   90-38128
                                       CIP

Printed in the United States of America
91 92 10 9 8 7 6 5 4 3

Dedicated to the thousands of men and women who have participated in the Kaiser Permanente FREEDOM FROM FAT® Program, Portland, Oregon.

Your comments and suggestions are reflected in each page of this book.

Thank You.

Comments, suggestions, or questions are welcome. Please send them to:

FREEDOM FROM FAT®
Kaiser Permanente
Department of Health Education and Health Promotion
7201 N. Interstate Avenue
Portland, Oregon 97217

CONTENTS

FOREWORD

We have all heard the messages loud and clear—"reduce fat to 30% of your total calories," "fats are fattening," "lose weight," "lower your cholesterol." We've heard it from the Surgeon General, food manufacturers, the American Heart Association, and our family physician. We read about the diet-fat connection in fashion and food magazines, newspapers, and in ads for weight loss programs.

But with all these recommendations and information, many people find it frustrating and time consuming to put these guidelines into practice. That's why we at Kaiser Permanente developed *Health Counts*—to help patients lower the fat in their diet the easy way. With *Health Counts* there is no "gramming" around. The usual grams of fat found on food labels are translated into calories. Fat calories, total calories, and percent calories from fat are listed for over 2,500 foods. Since fats have twice as many calories as do carbohydrates, a small reduction in fats can account for a bigger savings in calories.

Three Typical Health Counts *Users*

Mark has a family history of heart disease. His blood cholesterol level is 260 mg/dl. Mark's doctor told him to keep his daily fat intake to 30% of his total calories. Does this mean a life of tuna fish and carrot sticks?

Linda weighs 230 pounds. She is a "borderline" diabetic and has a family history of high blood pressure. Her nurse practitioner has given her a 1500 calorie diet. After 2 weeks she finds the diet boring. Does she have to stick to that one pre-planned diet or can she make up a more varied food plan at 1500 calories a day?

Megan is 20 pounds overweight. Each year she gains, loses, and regains. At 35 she is finding it harder to get the weight off. She fears she must either stay on a diet for he rest of her life, or face the fact that she will "end up a fat, dumpy lady!" Is there yet another possibility—maybe even a pleasant one?

Health Counts is a quick food counter reference for all the Marks and Lindas and Megans who need and want to make careful food choices. *Health Counts* takes all the guesswork and tedium out of counting fats and calories.

To keep his fat intake to 30%, Mark doesn't have to go on a tuna fish and carrot stick diet. His doctor said, "On an average, keep your total calories from fat to 30% of your daily calorie intake." If Mark keeps a record of everything he eats each day and looks up each item in *Health Counts*, he can quickly calculate his daily calories and what percent of those calories were from fat. In a couple of weeks, he will learn which foods are high in fat and which are low. He learns that he can indulge in occasional higher-fat foods because he plans well. For example, if he plans to eat a four-ounce T-bone steak for supper (trimmed, it's 43% fat), he might choose a very low-fat lunch so that his fat intake for the day is not over 30%. If he goes a little over 30% one day, however, he can make it up by choosing foods that are much lower in fat the next day. What's really important is his *weekly* percentage, not the percentage for one day only.

Linda checks with her nurse practitioner. She's told she doesn't really need a diet with pre-selected foods. She can select and prepare a variety of foods just as long as most of her choices are high in nutrients and together do not exceed the 1500 calorie limit. She can plan what she wants to eat for the next day, look up those foods in *Health Counts*, record the calorie count for each food item and then calculate the totals for the day. If her planned meals and snacks total more than 1500 calories for the day, she can plan to eat smaller portions or replace one or two foods with items that have fewer calories. *Health Counts* can help her do this quickly and accurately. As she learns to reduce her daily calories, Linda *will* lose weight—and she will also reduce her risk of developing high blood pressure and diabetes.

Megan doesn't have to face a future as a "fat lady." To understand her current eating patterns, Megan keeps a food diary. She records what she eats, how much, when, etc. Using *Health Counts*, she looks up and records the calories and calories from fat in each food she eats. After keeping records for two weeks, she can see which high-calorie foods she eats regularly. She may cut back on some of these and replace others with complex carbohydrates. (Complex carbohydrates, like pasta, bread and dried beans, are rich in nutrients and low in fats and calories.) Her food diary records show that she tends to get hungry each night around 9:30, so she checks out snacks in *Health Counts* and buys some low-calorie munchies. Lowering calories *without* exercise causes the body to lose lean muscle mass, not fat. Megan knows that she usually stays trim in the summer months when she is more active, but puts on almost a pound a week during the cold months when she is inactive. She realizes that to keep trim year round, she needs to make regular exercise a part of her year-round routine.

You will also come to realize that *it is important to eat more wisely.* This book will help you do the counting, record-keeping, and decision-making that spell success. In a day when diets, weight loss programs, and diet books proliferate, we feel confident that *Health Counts* is unmatched in helping you make low fat choices.

Judith Rossner, M.S., R.D.
FREEDOM FROM FAT®
Program Director

ACKNOWLEDGMENTS

Health Counts is the product of many people's efforts.

First published in 1983 under the title *Calorie Guide*, this first edition was developed for use in the **FREEDOM FROM FAT**® weight management program conducted by the Kaiser Permanente Center for Health Research in Portland, Oregon. It was designed to clearly show the fat content of commonly eaten foods and the high calorie impact fats have on one's diet. This was the work of Mitch Greenlick, Ph.D., director of the project, Shirley Craddick, R.D., Herman Frankel, M.D., Judith Rossner, M.S., R.D., and Victor Stevens, Ph.D.

Technical contributors include Dan Azevedo, Karen Crisp, R.D., Joyce Downing, Lois Drew, Sarah Frankel, Gillian Glass, John Hall, Judy Henderson, Robin Maxwell, Michael Rubino, Phyllis Snedeker, and Martie Sucec.

The *Calorie Guide* was revised and expanded in 1987 and was titled *Health Counts*. This production was supervised by Judith Rossner, M.S., R.D. The primary writer and graphic designer was Donna H. Dean, M.P.H. Luanna Squires, R.D. served as nutrition editor. Technical assistance was provided by Carolyn Studer, M.Ed., Kelly Johnson Streit, M.S., R.D., and Elizabeth Wagner, M.S. Production expertise was provided by Jim Anderson, Jennifer Boon, and Bruce Patten.

Health Counts: A Fat and Calorie Guide, the book you hold in your hands, is a significant improvement over earlier versions. Editor Luanna Squires, R.D. warrants special recognition for her extraordinary and diligent work in expanding and reorganizing the food tables. We are also appreciative of the technical assistance provided by Maggi Dorsett, M.S., R.D., Carol Mosman, R.D., Margaret Raker, M.S., R.D., and Robert Wilson, D.T.R. We are especially grateful to Donna H. Dean, M.P.H. for her creative writing skills in translating nutrition concepts into practical guidelines and suggestions.

There are scores of others we want to acknowledge. The work of many, many support and technical staff runs like a fiber through all these efforts. Special thanks to Becky Belangy, Linda Davis, George Tomberlin, and Ron Goldman.

Finally and fundamentally, management had confidence in our vision and backed it up. We are especially grateful to Ted Carpenter, Joy Gray, Mike Katcher, Ken Myers, and Al Weiland.

We also acknowledge the product and nutrient analysis provided by manufacturers represented in *Health Counts* and by Nutrition and Diet Services, Portland, Oregon.

Chapter 1

INTRODUCTION

Who Will Find this Book Useful?

Anyone who wants to make more thoughtful food choices.
You will find:

- The calorie and fat counts for over 2,500 foods.
- Practical guidelines and tools to help you make changes in your eating habits.
- A format that makes food items easy to find—and calorie and fat counting quick to do.

Food items are listed alphabetically *and* by food group. Food groups are:

CATEGORIES, such as fruits, meats, cookies, and beverages.

TYPES, such as Mexican or Oriental foods.

FOOD PRODUCTS or **RESTAURANTS**, such as Lean Cuisine or Arby's restaurant.

For example, you can turn to the McDonald's restaurant listing in the Food Group List and learn this about a typical fast food meal:

A Big Mac is	560 calories	and	292 calories	are from fat.
French Fries are	320 calories	and	154 calories	are from fat.
A Milkshake is	390 calories	and	95 calories	are from fat.
Totals:	1270 calories	and	541 calories	are from fat

Why so many calories in one quick meal? **FAT.** The kind of dietary fat that can also lead to hardening of the arteries, strokes and heart attacks.

The American Heart Association recommends that you cut back on the amount of fat in your diet. For most Americans, approximately 40% of daily calories are from fat! For a healthy heart 30% or less is best. Reducing your dietary fat will also help you control your weight, since fats, ounce for ounce, contain twice as many calories as protein or carbohydrates. Fat *is* fattening!

Look again at the fast food meal listed on page 1. In that one meal there are 541 calories from fat. How does that percentage of calories from fat compare to the recommended 30% or less? To calculate the percentage of calories from fat, divide the total calories from fat by the total calories in the meal. Like this:

$$\frac{\text{CALORIES FROM FAT}}{\text{TOTAL CALORIES IN THE MEAL}} \quad = \quad \frac{541}{1270} \quad = \quad 43\% \text{ FROM FAT}$$

What if you want to lower that percentage of fat to 30% or less? *Health Counts* can help you select a lower fat combination of foods. For example:

Turkey Sandwich and Soup:

Roast Turkey	3 ounces	150 calories	30	from fat
Rye Bread	2 slices	120 calories	a trace	from fat
Mayonnaise	1 tsp	33 calories	33	from fat
Lettuce	2 leaves	a trace	a trace	from fat
Tomato, fresh	3 slices	9 calories	a trace	from fat
Split Pea Soup	1 cup	145 calories	27	from fat
Apple (3 inch)	1	96 calories	8	from fat
	TOTALS:	553 calories	98	from fat

$$\frac{\text{CALORIES FROM FAT}}{\text{TOTAL CALORIES IN THE MEAL}} \quad = \quad \frac{98}{553} \quad = \quad 18\% \text{ FROM FAT}$$

Quite a difference from the fast-food meal! A difference *you* can make when you use *Health Counts*. A difference that—over the months and years—will make a significant impact on your ability to

- lose weight and keep it off
- maintain your ideal weight
- lower your blood cholesterol and therefore your risk of strokes and heart attacks
- lower your risk of developing diabetes and high blood pressure.

How do you change something as personal and important as eating habits? Over the past years, Kaiser Permanente researchers have developed a number of effective techniques and approaches. They have combined these techniques in a uniquely successful weight control program called Freedom from Fat®. The highlights of these techniques are summarized in the following sections:

- Keeping a Food Diary: Why and How
- Recommendations for Weight Management

- Cooking Tips: Cutting Down on Fat
- Calculating Calories and Fat in a Recipe
- Reading Food Labels

Keeping a Food Diary

Why Keep a Food Diary?

Recording what you eat and when you eat it may seem like an unnecessary nuisance at first. Kaiser Permanente research has shown, however, that those who kept four to five daily food diaries each week lost more weight than those who did not keep food diaries.

Recording what you eat and checking the calorie and fat count for each food tends to make you more thoughtful and less prone to automatic eating.

Your food diary is only a tool. Do not worry about trying to make it perfect. Simply use it to become more aware of what you eat and when you eat it. When you have kept a number of diaries, you will begin to see patterns and develop ideas about changes you wish to make.

How to Keep a Food Diary

A blank form you may reproduce for your own use is on pages 6–7. Take a look at it or make a copy now so you can follow these six steps:

1. Fill out the heading—both the date *and* the day of the week will be important when you begin to analyze your eating patterns. (Do I eat more on weekends, etc.?)

2. List everything you eat or drink immediately after each meal or snack so you do not forget it. Record:
   - the time you ate
   - what you ate
   - the amount (in standard measurements such as one cup, a tablespoon, one slice, etc.)
   - how it was prepared (fried, steamed, broiled, with butter, in oil, baked, etc.)

3. Look up each item in *Health Counts*, recall your serving size, calculate the total calories and calories from fat for a serving of that size and write

this down in the columns provided on the food diary form. For example, *Health Counts* lists:

FOOD		CALORIES		
	AMOUNT	TOTAL	FAT	%FAT
pork chop, top loin, broiled	1 oz	73	38	52

If you have a five-ounce chop, multiply the first two figures in the calories column by 5. Then record 365 in the total calories column and 190 in the calories from the fat column. (The percentage fat will be the same for five ounces as it is for one.)

So your food diary entry will look like this:

FOOD DIARY		DATE _June 27th_ DAY OF WEEK _Wed._		
TIME	AMOUNT	TYPE OF FOOD, BEVERAGE AND HOW PREPARED, INGREDIENTS	TOTAL CALORIES	CALORIES FROM FAT
8 pm	5 oz	Pork chop, top loin, broiled	365	190

4. At the end of the day, add up the total calories column and the calories from fat column. Then calculate the percentage of calories from fat for the entire day.

$$\frac{\text{TOTAL CALORIES FROM FAT}}{\text{TOTAL CALORIES}} = \text{PERCENTAGE CALORIES FROM FAT}$$

5. At the end of the week, review the totals from your daily food diaries. Then you can begin to see patterns—a skipped breakfast often followed by a high-fat mid-morning snack, a *very* low-calorie day ended with a 1500 calorie supper. After you summarize several weeks, you will clearly see patterns that need attention.

6. Analyze your eating patterns and plan the changes you want to make. The questions listed here will help you get started.

❏ Are your weekend days lower or higher in calories than weekdays?

❏ Do you compensate for extra high-calorie meals or days by lowering the calories in the next meal or day?

❏ How does day five compare with day one of your first week's diary? How does the second week's diary compare with the first week's?

❏ Are you beginning to eat smaller portions of those high-calorie foods you don't want to give up?

❏ Are you keeping your weekly percentage of calories from fat to 30% or less?

❏ Are you more conscious of automatic eating? What have you done about it?

❏ Do you tend to eat more in the evening if you have been too strict all day?

❏ If you are careful about what you eat, yet don't deprive yourself, does this have an effect on any tendency to binge?

❏ Are you keeping at least four to five diaries each week?

❏ Have you begun to replace high-fat meats with beans, fish, or poultry?

FOOD DIARY   DATE _____   DAY OF WEEK _____

TIME	AMOUNT	TYPE OF FOOD, BEVERAGE AND HOW PREPARED, INGREDIENTS	TOTAL CALORIES	CALORIES FROM FAT
		DAILY SUBTOTALS:		

TIME	AMOUNT	TYPE OF FOOD, BEVERAGE AND HOW PREPARED, INGREDIENTS	TOTAL CALORIES	CALORIES FROM FAT
		SUBTOTALS FROM PAGE 1:		
		DAILY SUBTOTALS:		

EXERCISE _____ FOR _____ MINUTES.   WEIGHT _____

PERCENTAGE OF CALORIES FROM FAT:

_____%

Recommendations for Weight Management

The difference between a fad or miracle diet and successful weight management is how you look one year later. Did you keep the weight off or regain it—and a bit more? Kaiser Permanente has helped thousands of men and women lose weight and keep it off. We share some of our successful techniques with you:

1. Keep your daily intake of calories from fat to 30% or less.

2. Gradually replace higher-fat foods with complex carbohydrates.
   - four or more vegetable servings and three or more fruit servings each day
   - five or more grain servings each day
   - one or more legume servings each week

3. Eat a variety of foods—vegetables, fruit, grains, dairy products, and protein—each day.

4. Keep five or more daily food diaries each week. These diaries help you see your eating patterns. Writing down what you eat and drink also makes you more committed to change and more aware of automatic eating.

5. If you are trying to lose weight:
   - Eat more frequently—3 to 6 times a day (meals and snacks)—in order to avoid the extreme hunger caused by long time periods between meals.
   - Exercise (continuous brisk walking, running, swimming or other aerobic activity) for at least 30 minutes, five times a week. This prevents burning your lean muscle mass instead of body fat as you cut down on calories.

The "No More Diets Plan"

The Formula: Fewer calories + lower weekly percentage of calories from fat + more exercise = weight loss + successful weight management.

Diets don't work. Diets help you lose weight—but not keep it off. Nobody wants to stay on a diet for life. A diet is something you go on and off. So your weight yo-yo's up and down. Diets make you feel deprived and angry. Diet is a four letter word.

Don't go on a diet. Don't even think of yourself as dieting. Learn to see yourself as "eating better" and "taking charge." Begin making the changes you want to make. (See the lists in Column A and Column B on pages 10–13.) As long as you keep the formula in mind and set weekly goals you can—and DO—reach, you will be moving toward success. Without a diet. Without guilt. And without feeling deprived.

Week One:

Select what you will do this week: one item from Column A and one item from Column B. Pick something you want to do. Something you are 85% sure you can and will do. Think about this:

- 3500 calories = 1 pound.
- 3500 calories less a week, with all else the same = 1 pound lost.
- 3500 calories less a week + 45-60 minutes of aerobic exercise 4 to 5 times a week = MORE weight loss.
- 3500 calories less a week + 30% or less calories from fat + 45 to 60 minutes of aerobic exercise 4 to 5 times a week = MOST weight loss.

Record your choices on your Weekly Check-Up form. (See pages 14–15.)

WARNING: Your total daily calories SHOULD NOT BE UNDER 1200 unless you are under the supervision of a physician.

Week Two:

Use your Weekly Check-Up form on page 14 to see how you did and to plan your next steps. How was it? Too easy? If so, aim a bit higher this week. (Then ask yourself, "Am I still 85% sure I can and will make it?")

If you didn't quite reach your goal, stick with it and think about cutting it down a bit. Maybe you tried to do too much. You know yourself and your abilities. Plan a bit more wisely this week.

Weeks Three, Four, Etc.:

Continue to build up your "collection of new skills" adding one or two a week from each column. *Remember to do what appeals to you.* That way you are more likely to do it.

You are not developing a "just-for-a-month" or "just-until-I-lose-20 pounds" plan. You are developing a way of eating you can make part of your life from now on! Give this time of *retraining yourself* the care and importance it deserves. And don't forget to give yourself the care and praise you deserve. You are doing very difficult and very important work. Your heart and arteries will thank you. Your family will thank you. You can add years of health and energy to your life.

Column A: Low-Fat Eating

1. Lower my weekly percentage of calories from fat by 5%.
   Lower my weekly percentage of calories from fat by 10%.
   Lower my weekly percentage of calories from fat by 15%.
   Lower my weekly percentage of calories from fat by 20%.
   Lower my weekly percentage of calories from fat by 25%.

2. Reduce my calories by 3500 this week.
   Reduce my calories by 4500 this week.
   Reduce my calories by 5500 this week.
   Reduce my calories by 6500 this week.
   Reduce my calories by 7500 this week.

3. Eat five or six smaller meals instead of 2 or 3 big ones each day.

4. Keep a food diary 2 days this week. (See "Keeping A Food Diary" on pages 3–5.)
   Keep a food diary 3 days this week.
   Keep a food diary 4 days this week.
   Keep a food diary 5 or more days this week.

5. Introduce 2 new low-fat foods into my eating this week.

6. Purge my kitchen/house/desk/car of high-fat, high-sugar temptations.

7. Eat low-fat snacks, instead of high-fat or high-sugar ones, once or twice each day.

8. Select or prepare 1 or 2 low-fat quick meals this week instead of the "fast food" solutions that are high in fat and sugar.

9. Once this week choose beans, fish or skinned poultry instead of a red-meat entree.

10. Eat 1 or 2 more vegetables this week.
    Eat 1 or 2 more vegetables each day.
    Eat at least 4 servings of vegetables every day.

11. Eat 1 or 2 more pieces of fresh fruit this week.
    Eat one or more pieces of fresh fruit each day.
    Eat at least 3 pieces of fresh fruit each day.

12. Eat 1 or 2 more servings of bread, pasta and rice this week.

    Eat 1 or 2 more servings of bread, pasta and rice each day.

    Eat 5 or more servings of bread, pasta and rice each day.

13. Reduce the fat in my food preparation by using the "Cooking Tips: Cutting Down on Fat" (on pages 16–17) 1 time this week.

    Reduce the fat in my food preparation by using these cooking tips 1 time a day.

    Reduce the fat in my food preparation by using these cooking tips every time I prepare food.

14. Eat a smaller portion of red meat or cheese 2 times this week.

    Eat a smaller portion of red meat or cheese each time I choose them.

    Substitute a lower-fat choice for red meat or cheese 1 time this week.

    Substitute a lower-fat choice of red meat or cheese 1 time each day.

Column B: Management Tools

All the changes in the world from COLUMN A will not help you develop the skills to manage your own weight! You need COLUMN B for that.

Exercise

1. Add 5 minutes to my current aerobic exercise schedule. (See "Exercise: The Secret Weapon" on page 16.)

    Add 10 minutes to my current aerobic exercise schedule.

    Add 20 minutes to my current aerobic exercise schedule.

    Add 30 minutes to my current aerobic exercise schedule.

    Add 45 minutes to my current aerobic exercise schedule.

2. Exercise 1 more day this week.

    Exercise 2 more days this week.

    Exercise 3 more days this week.

    Exercise 4 more days this week.

    Exercise 5 more days this week.

    Exercise 6 more days this week.

3. Increase my walking speed until I reach the level of exertion where I am pushed but still able to hold a conversation without getting breathless.

Support Network

1. Ask one person (from family, work, friends) to help support my weight loss efforts.

2. Talk to my support person at least 1 time a week, discussing progress and problems.

3. Ask another person from another area of my life to support my efforts and be available to talk with me.

4. Talk with each of my two support people at least 1 time a week.

5. Call my support people when/if I get discouraged, tempted to binge or give up. (I will reach for the handle on the telephone instead of the handle on the refrigerator!)

6. Begin my chats with support people on a positive note, "This is what I have done for myself this week."

7. Share my food diary with my support people. Practice receiving their praise with a simple "Thank you." (I am getting used to feeling good about myself!)

Managing and Problem-Solving

1. Set two goals—one in Column A, one in Column B—for the week. Then ask myself, "Is each goal big enough to matter and small enough to achieve?" If not, I'll adjust it.

2. Keep track of my weight and exercise time each day.

3. Take my body measurements and record them at one time during the week.

4. Using my food diary records, keep track of my daily calories and percentage of calories from fat.

5. Review my records once a week to check my progress and re-plan as needed. (Use the Check-Up form on page 14.)

6. Avoid 1 tempting situation to eat "my old high-fat favorites" this week. (See "Dealing with Triggers," pages 26–28.)

Self-Image and Self-Esteem

1. Encourage myself by positive self-talk 1 or 2 times a day.

    For example:

    > "I'm getting better and better at choosing low-fat foods."

    > "I have the ability to give up negative thoughts and replace them with a positive attitude."

    > "It feels good to be taking care of myself."

2. Ask one of my support people to help when I'm discouraged by reminding me to also look at what *I have* accomplished.

3. Look at my food diary and weight records and use the progress I see to encourage myself. *"Look how far I've come!"*

4. Practice letting a slip or setback be just that—a temporary thing—not a catastrophe or a judgement on my ability.

Preventing a Binge

1. I won't deprive myself and get "starved." I'll eat 5 or 6 smaller meals spread throughout the day. (See "The Fine Art of Grazing" and "How to Pick Yourself Up" on pages 24–25.)

3. When I'm hungry for a snack, I'll eat a high-energy food like fruit or a muffin. I know a candy bar or high-sugar food will only give me a quick rush that's followed by an even deeper energy slump.

4. I'll avoid the dieter's trap of skipping meals. I know this only sets me up to feel I deserve more at the next meal.

5. When I feel hungry, I will wait a few minutes and not eat automatically. As I wait, I'll check in with myself: Am I really hungry for food—or maybe for company or comfort?

    If I find my hunger is emotional, I'll either reach out to another for company or comfort, or meet that need myself in a nonfattening way.

MY WEEKLY CHECK-UP

Directions: Write down your choices and track your progress weekly.

Week 1

Column A (1 choice)

My choice: _____
_____
_____

Mastered? ❑ Yes ❑ Not quite

Comments: _____

Decision: ❑ Keep working on it ❑ Mastered, select new goal

Column B (1 choice)

My choice: _____
_____
_____

Mastered? ❑ Yes ❑ Not quite

Comments: _____

Decision: ❑ Keep working on it ❑ Mastered, select new goal

Week 2

Column A (1 or 2 choices)

My choice: _____
_____
_____

Mastered? ❑ Yes ❑ Not quite

Comments: _____

Decision: ❑ Keep working on it ❑ Mastered, select new goal

Column B (1 or 2 choices)

My choice: _____
_____
_____

Mastered? ❑ Yes ❑ Not quite

Comments: _____

Decision: ❑ Keep working on it ❑ Mastered, select new goal

MY WEEKLY CHECK-UP

(Make copies of this form for your next weeks before you begin to use it.)

Week __

Column A (1 or 2 choices)

My choice: _____

_____

_____

Mastered? ❑ Yes   ❑ Not quite

Comments: _____

Decision: ❑ Keep working on it ❑ Mastered, select new goal

Column B (1 or 2 choices)

My choice: _____

_____

_____

Mastered? ❑ Yes   ❑ Not quite

Comments: _____

Decision: ❑ Keep working on it ❑ Mastered, select new goal

Week __

Column A (1 or 2 choices)

My choice: _____

_____

_____

Mastered? ❑ Yes   ❑ Not quite

Comments: _____

Decision: ❑ Keep working on it ❑ Mastered, select new goal

Column B (1 or 2 choices)

My choice: _____

_____

_____

Mastered? ❑ Yes   ❑ Not quite

Comments: _____

Decision: ❑ Keep working on it ❑ Mastered, select new goal

Exercise: The Secret Weapon

*"If you could sell a drug that would help people lose weight, slow the aging process, prevent a heart attack, and increase self esteem, you'd make a fortune. But the miracle cure already exists, and it is not in the shape of a pill. It is exercise, and it can work those wonders and more."**

"Who wouldn't jump at the opportunity to eat more and weigh less? People who exercise vigorously do just that" according to a number of studies. Exercise changes the way the body burns and stores calories. In fact, when you exercise, *you continue to burn more calories for hours afterwards.*

Studies also report that exercise makes people "cheerier, more self-reliant, and less anxious."**

What kind of exercise does all this? *Aerobic exercise. Exercise that is continuous, moderate, and frequent.* Walking is one of the best forms of aerobic exercise. You need no special place, time or talent, and it is very inexpensive.

To get started, walk (or take up a similar exercise) for at least five minutes this week.

Making *small* changes is essential for success. If you start out with a demanding exercise program, most likely you'll soon get discouraged and discontinue it. Small changes, however, easily fit into your daily routine. Gradually, you will increase your exercise time. For now, make it moderate and take it easy. *Simply get moving!*

Without exercise, you cannot lose weight and keep it off. Select one or two of the many excellent books on exercise and use it as an inspiration guide.

Cooking Tips: Cutting Down on Fat

1. Reduce fat in recipes by 1/3 to 1/2.

2. Before cooking, trim excess fat from meat and remove skin from poultry.

3. Cool soups and stews in the refrigerator. Skim fat before reheating to serve.

4. Whenever possible, use low-fat products and cooking methods. See the table on the next page.

*"Exer-guide, A Look at the Benefits of Exercise" by Bonnie Liebman, *NUTRITION ACTION*, November, 1981, pages 9–11. Center for Science in the Public Interest (CSPI) Washington, D.C.

For	Substitute	Calories Saved
1 cup whole milk	1 cup skim milk	76
	1 cup 1% milk	59
1 cup whole milk ricotta cheese	1 cup 2% low-fat cottage cheese	224
	1 cup regular cottage cheese	194
	1 cup part-skim ricotta cheese	90
1 cup heavy cream	1 cup skim evaporated milk	648
	1 cup regular evaporated milk	508
1 cup sour cream	1 cup plain low-fat yogurt	355
	1 cup blended 2% low-fat cottage cheese	289
1 cup regular mayonnaise	1 cup plain low-fat yogurt	1460
	1/2 cup plain low-fat yogurt with 1/2 cup regular mayonnaise	870
	1 cup reduced calorie mayonnaise	800
1 cup whole milk white sauce with 2 Tbsp flour and 2 Tbsp of butter	1 cup white sauce made with 1% white milk, 2 Tbsp flour and no fat	263
1 oz cheddar cheese	1 oz low-fat processed cheese	42
	2 Tbsp grated parmesan cheese	62
1/4 cup regular margarine or butter	1/4 cup diet margarine	208
2 large whole eggs	1/2 cup low-cholesterol egg substitute	54
1 large whole egg	2 egg whites	41
1 cup condensed cream soup	1 cup white sauce made with skim milk, 1 Tbsp flour and no fat	80
6 1/2 oz can oil-packed tuna	6 1/2 oz can water-packed tuna	123
Mayonnaise or sour cream based sauces, dips and dressings	vinegar, mustard, tomato juice or fat-free bouillon base	*
Fried meat	broil, bake, or roast on rack or microwave	*
Browned meat	non-stick pan—no added fat	*
Stir-fried meat	"stir-steam" in water rather than oil	*

* Because food quantities are not specified, calories saved cannot be calculated.

Calculating Calories and Fat in a Recipe

1. List all ingredients and amounts.

2. Look up total calories and calories from fat for each ingredient. Calculate the new totals as shown in the example below.

   Refried Beans
   1 cup = 248 calories − 16 calories from fat
   2 cups = 496 calories − 32 calories from fat

BEAN BURRITOS

serves: 4

INGREDIENTS		CALORIES	
		TOTAL	FAT
2c	canned refried beans	496	32
1/2	medium onion	19	tr
1 tsp	garlic	—	—
	pepper to taste	—	—
	chili powder	—	—
8	corn tortillas	504	40
	4 SERVINGS:	1019	72
	1 SERVING:	255	18

3. Add up the total calories column and the calories from fat column.

4. Divide the totals by the number of servings:

$$\frac{1019}{4} = 255 \qquad \frac{72}{4} = 18$$

Reading Food Labels

Quite often, the nutritional information you find on labels is in the form of grams. It is easy to convert grams to calories. The following table shows how many calories are in each gram of:

	GRAMS	CALORIES
Carbohydrate	1	4
Protein	1	4
Fat	1	9
Alcohol	1	7

One gram of fat has over twice as many calories as a gram of carbohydrate or a gram of protein. For this reason, you can easily be misled when reading labels. Look at this carrot cake mix label for example:

Portion size, 1/12 of package without frosting	
Calories	330
Protein (grams)	4
Carbohydrates (grams)	40
Fat (grams)	17

To convert the grams into calories, do some simple multiplication. If 1 gram of fat is equal to 9 calories, then 17 grams would be 9 times 17 or 153 calories.

Fat	9×17 grams	= 153 calories
Protein	4×4 grams	= 16 calories
Carbohydrates	4×40 grams	= 160 calories
	TOTAL	= 329 calories

You will notice that the label said 330 calories and your total is 329. This is because fractions of a gram are "rounded off" to the nearest number. On some labels the difference between the label total and the one you calculate will be even greater. Don't let it concern you. Use your own calculations. Your figures will be accurate enough.

Begin Right Now!

Don't put it off. Take the blank food diary form on pages 6–7 and reproduce several copies. Write down what you've eaten so far today. For breakfast. For mid-morning snack. For lunch. Describe each item as well as you can. How big was the danish pastry? Were the potatoes you had for lunch fried, mashed, with or without gravy? Write it all down and then look up each item in *Health Counts*. Note three figures—total calories, calories from fat, and percentage of calories from fat. What kind of totals do you have for the day so far? Surprised? What is your percentage of calories from fat? Thirty percent or less? (The formula for calculating percentage of calories from fat is on page 4.)

In a few days, you will have enough information in your food diary to begin looking for patterns you will want to change. Focus on one change at a time. Make small changes. Changes you can easily fit into your life. Small, easy changes add up. They become new habits. Healthy habits that last. Habits that show—*your health counts*.

Chapter 2

FACTS AND TIPS

Understanding Cholesterol

If you are overweight, most likely your daily calorie intake is 40% or more fat. For most Americans that means they are eating a great deal of saturated fat and cholesterol. If your diet is high in fat and cholesterol, no matter what your family history or current blood cholesterol level—you are probably clogging up your arteries.

Cholesterol is a fat-like substance. The cholesterol you eat in eggs and red meat, for example, raises the level of cholesterol in your blood. But, even more importantly, the amounts and kinds of *fats* you eat affect your blood cholesterol level.

Saturated fat, *more than cholesterol,* can raise blood cholesterol levels. Polyunsaturated fats and monounsaturated fats help to lower blood or serum cholesterol, but not enough to overcome the disadvantages of a high-fat diet.

Although you may inherit a tendency for elevated blood cholesterol, *you can greatly influence your cholesterol level by diet and exercise.* Each 1-percent decrease in cholesterol is associated with a 2-percent decline in heart attack risk.

To control your cholesterol level, a low-fat, high-fiber eating plan is best. You need not make a production out of "watching for high cholesterol foods." *It's almost impossible to get too much cholesterol or saturated fat if you manage to keep your total calories from fat down to 25-30%.*

You have probably heard the expressions, "good cholesterol" and "bad cholesterol." These terms refer to blood fats called lipoproteins. Lipoproteins carry cholesterol through the blood. HDL (high-density lipoproteins) are good because they carry cholesterol away from body tissues. LDL (low-density lipoproteins) are not good because they dump cholesterol in the vessels. Over time these deposits grow thick and can clog or close the vessel. When the clogged vessel is in the brain, a stroke occurs. When the clogged vessel is in the heart, angina or a heart attack may strike.

So what choices should you make for your 25–30% fat? Avoid saturated fats, use polyunsaturated fats by preference, and occasionally use monounsaturated fats to flavor or season a dish (see the definitions of these fats on page 22).

SATURATED FATS are solid at room temperature. They are found in most animal products *and in some vegetable products*. The more saturated the fat, the harder it will be at room temperature. When reading labels, watch for saturated fats. Even if the label says, "contains no cholesterol," the product may be high in saturated vegetable fats. Some common saturated vegetable fats are: coconut oil, palm oil, cocoa butter, hydrogenated fats, and oils. *Products with these oils will add to your cholesterol problem just as surely as the fat in red meat, eggs or cheese.* Examples of other foods with saturated fats are: chocolate, deep-fried foods, like chicken and french fries, corn and potato chips, pastries, and ice cream.

UNSATURATED FATS are the ones to choose. They have no cholesterol. They also help you lower your current blood cholesterol level. These friendly fats come in two basic kinds: polyunsaturated and monounsaturated.

POLYUNSATURATED FATS are your best friends in the fat family. *They are highly unsaturated.* Examples of products with the highest concentration of polyunsaturated fats are: safflower, sunflower, and corn oils and the margarines made from them.

MONOUNSATURATED FATS are *slightly unsaturated*. Canola oil, peanut oil, olive oil, and avocados are examples of monounsaturated fats.

Beware and be wise. Fats, whether they raise or lower cholesterol, add calories and pounds. To lose weight and be cholesterol-conscious, *avoid saturated fats and use only small amounts of poly- and monounsaturated fats for flavoring and cooking.* The whole idea is less is best!

Cutting Down the Clog

Know your blood cholesterol level and if possible, keep it below the recommended 200 mg. level.

What Do the Numbers Mean?

Desirable	199 mg/dl or less
Borderline high	200-239 mg/dl
High	240 mg/dl or more

1. Keep your percentage of calories from fat down to 25–30% a week. Use your food diary to check this.
2. Cut down on saturated fats. (See page 23 for more on saturated fats.)
3. Increase the good (HDL) and lower the bad (LDL) cholesterol by eating a low-fat, high-fiber diet and by exercising regularly.

4. Limit your dietary cholesterol to 300 mg. or less a day.

5. Shed those excess pounds. (You *will*—if you keep to your exercise and low-fat, high-fiber program!)

6. If you smoke, stop.

A change in diet is still the primary way to lower cholesterol. But the emphasis has shifted from limiting dietary cholesterol to limiting total fat.

Fat Saturation Table

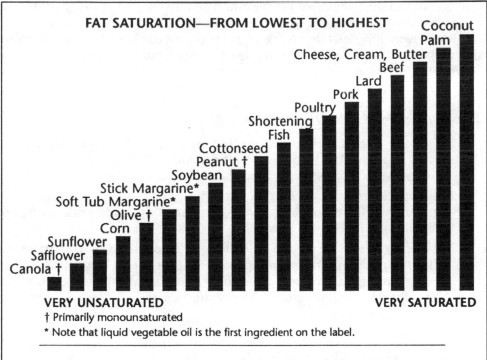

FAT SATURATION—FROM LOWEST TO HIGHEST

Coconut
Palm
Cheese, Cream, Butter
Beef
Lard
Pork
Poultry
Shortening
Fish
Cottonseed
Peanut †
Soybean
Stick Margarine*
Soft Tub Margarine*
Olive †
Corn
Sunflower
Safflower
Canola †

VERY UNSATURATED   VERY SATURATED

† Primarily monounsaturated
* Note that liquid vegetable oil is the first ingredient on the label.

A SPECIAL NOTE ABOUT MEAT AND DAIRY PRODUCT LABELS

Percentage fat labels on all meat and dairy products are by weight and not by calories. Keep this in mind or you will find yourself misled.

A turkey bologna, for example, that is labeled 80% fat free, is not as lean as you might think. The 20% fat noted on this label is 20% of the weight, not the calories. When you calculate the percentage of calories from fat, you discover it is 72%—not 20%!

Your best buy for a low-fat meat product is one labeled 95% or more lean.

The Fine Art of Grazing

Your body was designed to eat small amounts of food several times a day. Avoid the afternoon slump and the evening binge by grazing. Eat several smaller meals and planned snacks throughout the day.

You need a good breakfast to refuel after a night's sleep. Then, throughout the day, you need periodic refueling.

Your body is more like a washing machine that runs on quarters than your car which you can fuel up once and run for hundreds of miles. *You can't put in $10.00 and expect it to run all day without problems.* When you overeat your body promptly converts the overload into fat. On the other hand, if you skip breakfast, skimp on lunch or snack on jelly doughnuts or candy bars—*your body runs out of quarters.* Some people become tired, distracted, moody or drowsy and crave sweets or caffeine to give them a pick up.

Both overeating *and* depriving yourself throw the body's energy rhythm out of whack. Then, when evening comes and your resistance is low, you begin the "long snack" that can easily become a binge.

To avoid the evening binge—and the afternoon slump—work *with* your body's energy needs. *Complex carbohydrates provide your body with a steady supply of energy like a time-release capsule.*

1. Learn to graze. Eat five or six smaller meals spaced throughout the day. Eat a good breakfast, cut back a bit on your lunch and dinner, and use these saved calories for planned snacks.

2. Eat more complex carbohydrates. They are high-energy foods that gradually release nutrients and help your body avoid wide swings in blood sugar levels.

3. Avoid foods high in fat and refined sugar. These foods set you up for the afternoon slump and evening binge. Fats required large amounts of energy for digestion. Sugar gives you a quick but short-lived energy that does little to meet long-term energy needs.

How to Pick Yourself Up

When you seem to be bottoming out on the energy scale, these simple steps will help you build up steam again. Complex carbohydrates provide your body with a steady supply of energy like a time-release capsule.

1. Eat *energy foods—complex carbohydrates.* Begin with a hearty breakfast. This good start sets you up to feel good and to continue making wise

choices during the day. Choose from whole grain cereals and bread, bagels, muffins, fresh fruit, and low-fat or non-fat milk or yogurt.

2. Prevent energy slumps during the day. Avoid sugar highs. Don't wait until you are starved to eat. Plan energy snacks mid-morning and mid-afternoon before you get tired or hungry. Energy snacks like fresh fruit, pretzels, popcorn, bagels, and low fat crackers are tasty, filling, and are essentially fat free!

3. Drink at least 2 quarts of water a day. Water helps flush and freshen your body system.

4. Get back into your regular exercise program. *Exercise—even when you are tired—gives you energy.*

5. Listen to your body and respect what it tells you. Is your energy gauge at low or near empty?

6. Review your schedule. What can you get rid of, postpone, or delegate? Set more reasonable limits. Practice saying "No."

HIGH-ENERGY MUFFINS
yields: 12 muffins

INGREDIENTS

2 cups	All-Bran cereal
1/2 cup	molasses
1-1/2 cups	skim milk
1	egg
1 cup	flour
1 teaspoon	soda

Add All-Bran to the molasses and milk. Soak for 15 minutes. Beat the egg and add it to the bran mixture. Sift flour and soda together and add to the bran. Fill slightly oiled tins 2/3-full. Bake at 350 degrees for about 20 minutes.

PER SERVING

Calories	115
Calories from Fat	9
% Calories from Fat	8

Dealing with Triggers

Everyone knows that once you pull the trigger it's too late for second thoughts. So it is with triggers to eat. Triggers set off automatic eating. You pass the ice cream store and you say, "One single-dip cone won't hurt that much..." You pull in and order your favorite. Maybe you order a double dip once you get inside and the anticipation takes over.

It is much easier to deal with whatever triggers you to eat than it is to deal with the eating itself once the urge takes over. Deal successfully with your triggers and you will have fewer urges to eat inappropriately. Less need to rely on will power to keep you on track.

Use your food diary to record where you were and what else you were doing at the time. As you become more aware of situations that trigger eating you can change automatic eating into planned eating—or—no eating at all!

To successfully manage triggers:

1. Avoid the triggers.
2. Scramble the trigger situation.
3. Respond to the trigger in a new way.

Avoid the Trigger

Avoidance is the easiest and most effective approach. Does passing the dough-nut shop on the way home from work each evening trigger an urge to pull in for "just one"? Try driving home by a different route.

Scramble the Trigger Situation

Break the link between the trigger and eating by disrupting the trigger pattern. Does coming home trigger you to go straight to the refrigerator for a snack? Try changing or scrambling your routine. Come in a different door. Go directly to a different room in the house. Rearrange the furniture in your living room. Sit in a different chair—not the one you usually sit in when you think, "I wonder what I could have for a snack?"

Respond in a New Way

Do television commercials trigger you to head for a snack? Try substituting another behavior during commercials—one that you can't do while eating. Needlework. Stretching or in-place exercises.

Use the boxed questions that follow as a worksheet. Plan ahead. How will you manage those dangerous triggers? It takes practice to change habits built up over a lifetime. Study your food diary. As you identify more situations that are triggers for you, *use and reuse the worksheet.* You don't get to be "in charge" without doing your homework!

Feelings as Triggers

Feelings can be powerful triggers to eat. Your mood often dictates when you eat and what you eat. You're on the way home from work tired and hungry and want a no-fuss meal, so you drive into McDonald's. Or—you celebrate a job well done and reach for that gooey brownie.

Through the years most of us have learned to link emotional feelings and food. Very often we are feeding our emotional feelings, not our physical hunger.

Knowing this gives us power. We can find other ways to "feed our feelings" that do not put on pounds—and we don't have to go hungry to do it.

As you record what you eat in your food diary also jot down what you were feeling. How were you feeling when you began to snack? *Is eating your automatic response to certain feelings?* Now, use the worksheet following these comments. Are certain feelings triggers to eat? How could you manage this better? Plan some new approaches now to have ready when the trigger pulls back.

As you break the link between feelings and food you will be amazed at your own power to take charge of your life. And you will be well on the way to *becoming free from fat.*

Managing Triggers

How do Triggers Work?

As simply as 1, 2, 3.

- Look over my food diary.
- Pick two times I ate when I wish I had not...

3 *How did I feel afterwards?*

1 *What was the trigger?*

2 *What did I do?*

How Can I Manage Triggers Better?

- **Avoid the trigger if possible.** This is your strongest defense. If your trigger is a *combination* of coming home when you are tired and hungry, you can't avoid coming home. But you can avoid coming home *tired and hungry.* Do some relaxation exercises to refresh yourself before you leave for home. Or snack on some fresh fruit, wash your face and freshen up to avoid the combination of events that triggers you to eat.

- **Scramble the trigger situation.** Change the coming-home experience. Disrupt the old patterns. Come in a different door. Have no food in sight in the kitchen. Or openly enjoy a low-fat snack and feel proud of yourself rather than sneaky and guilty.

- **Respond to the trigger in a new way.** This is the most difficult approach. Filling the emptiness with a new response is, however, powerful. Most often it works best when you *combine* it with avoiding triggers and scrambling trigger situations. A new response to one of your eating triggers might be to take a walk, brush your teeth or take a quick shower to refresh yourself. Also try relaxing with deep-breathing exercises or stretching. Take a nap. Make a cup of tea and sip it slowly.

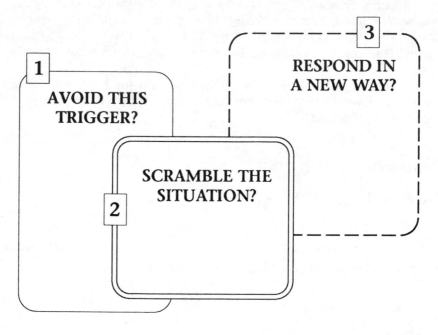

1 AVOID THIS TRIGGER?

2 SCRAMBLE THE SITUATION?

3 RESPOND IN A NEW WAY?

GETTING STARTED

How the Secret Weapon Works

Exercise—the secret weapon—changes the way your body burns and stores fat. If you take in fewer calories and burn more, you lose weight. Exercise trains your body to burn calories at its best level.

Getting the right balance between calories-in and calories-burned is tricky. Each person differs. Some need more calories than others. Some burn calories more efficiently.

We all need approximately 1200 or more calories a day for energy and to re-build tissue. As you go below 1200 calories, you increase the likelihood that your body will have to tear down lean muscle and organ tissue for energy. You'll lose weight—but *you can also seriously damage the very muscles you count on to burn off excess fat. When you do this, you also slow down your metabolism and make it even harder to burn calories for energy rather than store them as fat.*

Here's where the secret weapon comes in. Exercise trains your body to burn calories at its best level. Not only while you are exercising but for many hours afterwards. When you exercise regularly, you are building a lean, efficient body machine. And you don't have to starve yourself!

On the other hand, dieting without exercise prompts your body to shut down its fat-burning furnaces. *Dieting alone won't work.* Not for long. You may lose weight, but that weight loss is primarily water and muscle tissue. As soon as the diet is over, you'll regain the weight you lost and often more. And the weight you regain is all fat!

The formula for losing a pound a week is simple. *Five hundred fewer calories each day.* Eat a bit less and burn a bit more! For example—Sue usually takes in 2000 calories a day. If she cuts that back by 300 calories daily and walks for 30 to 45 minutes—4 to 5 times a week—she could lose a pound or more in a week.

Individual weight loss varies quite a bit. *Consider these figures as an example more than a standard to measure yourself by.* The secret is to cut back on some calories—especially fat calories—and burn more—through exercise.

Start today. Remember—to lose weight, your exercise must be:

- Continuous—no stops and starts—keep moving.
- Moderate—a good pace, but not so hard you get winded.
- Regular—4 to 5 times a week.

Put your secret weapon to work.

Goal Setting: The Ladder of Success

Goal setting is a powerful management tool. You build a ladder of success. One step at a time.

You break down huge, overwhelming tasks into small, concrete goals you can easily reach. As you reach each step, you feel proud and successful. You are encouraged to take the next step. It's easy. Your confidence builds. You keep moving. How do you begin?

First, set your long-term goal or direction. Where do you want to go? For example, your direction might be:

- I want to lose ___ pounds.
- I want to wear size ___ dress or suit.
- I want to exercise for 45-60 minutes—4 or 5 times a week.
- I want to lower my percentage of calories from fat to 25%.
- I want to keep 5 food diaries each week.
- I want to reduce my blood cholesterol level.

Next, select some small steps or short-term goals that lead in that direction. Then ask yourself:

- Is this something I will *do,* not what I will avoid?
- Can I actually *see* it—so I'll know when I've done it?
- *Is it reachable*—"Are my chances of success 85% or better?" If the answer is "No," re-work your goal or choose another more reachable one.

When the steps are reachable, you succeed each week. You are able to make plans and follow through with them. Little by little, success by success, you come into your own power. In the end, you will be able to successfully take on any task, no matter how awesome, because you can break it down into manageable steps.

Self-Esteem and Self-Talk

Sometimes we get into a place where it is difficult to feel good about ourselves. Our society tells us we should be as slender as a model. You never see an overweight person draped around a new Porsche as a sales come-on. Messages telling us we are not OK bombard us from every side. And we buy those messages—at a great price to our self-esteem.

Then we take those messages inside and begin to send them to ourselves. Listen to what you say to yourself. How much of it is negative? How often during one hour do you put yourself down or judge yourself? And then—you put yourself down for putting yourself down. And on it goes. This habit—and it is a habit—eats away at your self-esteem and self-confidence. But it's only a habit—you can change it!

You can learn to manage your self-talk just as surely as you learn to manage any behavior. The techniques are the same.

Why bother? To become your own best friend. Someone who will love you and support you no matter what.

Positive Self-Talk

If you listen, you will hear a nearly continuous "inner conversation" going on in your mind.

The mind is busy talking to itself about life, feelings, other people, oneself. . . . *You can use these thoughts to help change your behavior.* Your thoughts are powerful. They influence your body, your feelings, your emotions, and your behavior. In fact, you *become* what you *tell yourself you are.*

Letting Go of Negative Thoughts

Experts say that most people spend 70% of their waking time in negative thoughts and self-criticism. No wonder we feel drained at the end of the day.

Positive Affirmations

Affirmations are an excellent way to replace or contradict negative thoughts that discourage you or hold you back. An affirmation is a positive, encouraging statement you make to yourself. For example, you might say to yourself as you walk: "Getting slimmer. Getting trimmer. Better cookin'. Better lookin'."

Some guidelines:

1. Make it a "now" statement—not a future one. Say it as if it already exists.
2. Make it as positive as you can. Say what you want, not what you don't want.
3. Make it personal. With special meaning for you. One that contradicts an old negative "self-talk tape" you've been playing far too long.
4. Repeat your affirmations many times a day: on waking, while you brush your teeth, as you wait for the elevator, or in the lunch line, while sitting at a red light, just before you go to sleep at night....
5. Write, print or type your affirmations on a piece of paper and paste them on a mirror, your car dashboard, the telephone—anywhere you might see them often during the day.

Some examples:

"I am getting better and better at choosing lower fat foods."

"I am taking care of myself by exercising regularly."

"I have the ability to refuse to paticipate in self destructive behaviors."

"I am kind and compassionate with myself."

"I am dealing constructively with my irritations without eating."

"I am asking for what I want instead of stuffing my feelings with food."

"I am creating a nurturing and supportive network of friends."

Social Support

People can support or sabotage your efforts to change your eating habits and take up regular exercise. To manage your program, build a strong support system to help you make and maintain changes.

The support of others is a powerful influence because it often provides immediate rewards. "Honey, I'm proud of you. You went right out for your walk as soon as you got home tonight!" Your glow lasts all evening. And you are more likely to walk again the next night after work. You are beginning to change. Develop a cluster of friends at work and at home who are especially interested in your progress.

- Select those who want to help you succeed and ask them if they will meet with you regularly.

- Find some supporters both at work and at home.
- Listen to their remarks and ask them for ideas about overcomming barriers.
- Let them in on your long-term goals and ask them to help you keep moving in the right direction.
- Welcome their encouragement—you'll be building a warmer world around you!

Fat Is Fattening

The average American's basic three square meals a day are over-rich in fat. Almost half of our daily calories are from fat.

For a healthy heart, the American Heart Association recommends you cut back dietary fat to 30%. Less fat in your meals will also help you control you weight. Fats, ounce for ounce, contain twice as many calories as protein or carbohydrates. Fat is fattening.

Fat is also sneaky. It hides in many foods: meats, dairy products, nuts, seeds, sauces, salad dressings, pastries, desserts, and mayonnaise. You know how to be wary of sugar. You have not yet learned to be "fat detectives." You have to *look for it* to find fat and lower your daily percentage.

You do have a helper. Complex carbohydrates. *You can win the calories battle by substituting complex carbohydrates for fat.* Complex carbohydrates are much lower in both fat content and calories. For example, a large serving of pasta is filling, inexpensive, lower in fat and has fewer calories than a small serving of pork chops.

Your second helper is this book. As you plan your meal, check to see how many calories each food contains. Note the percentage of calories from fat in each food. If the fat percentage is high, consider substituting another food or lowering the fat content in that food.

High-Fat and Low-Fat Meals

On the next 8 pages you can practice being a "fat detective." Compare the fat and calorie content of some high-fat and low-fat meals. The first 4 pages show the amount of fat in these meals and the second four pages show the calorie content of the same meals.

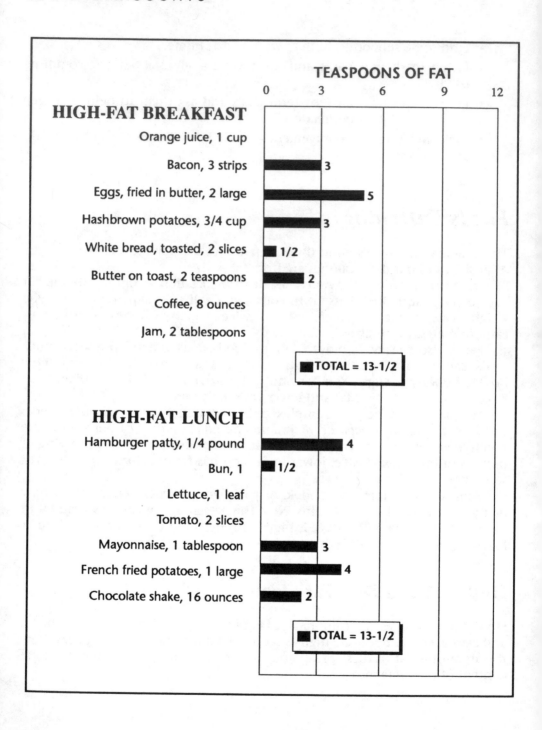

TEASPOONS OF FAT

0   3   6   9   12

HIGH-FAT BREAKFAST

Orange juice, 1 cup

Bacon, 3 strips — 3

Eggs, fried in butter, 2 large — 5

Hashbrown potatoes, 3/4 cup — 3

White bread, toasted, 2 slices — 1/2

Butter on toast, 2 teaspoons — 2

Coffee, 8 ounces

Jam, 2 tablespoons

TOTAL = 13-1/2

HIGH-FAT LUNCH

Hamburger patty, 1/4 pound — 4

Bun, 1 — 1/2

Lettuce, 1 leaf

Tomato, 2 slices

Mayonnaise, 1 tablespoon — 3

French fried potatoes, 1 large — 4

Chocolate shake, 16 ounces — 2

TOTAL = 13-1/2

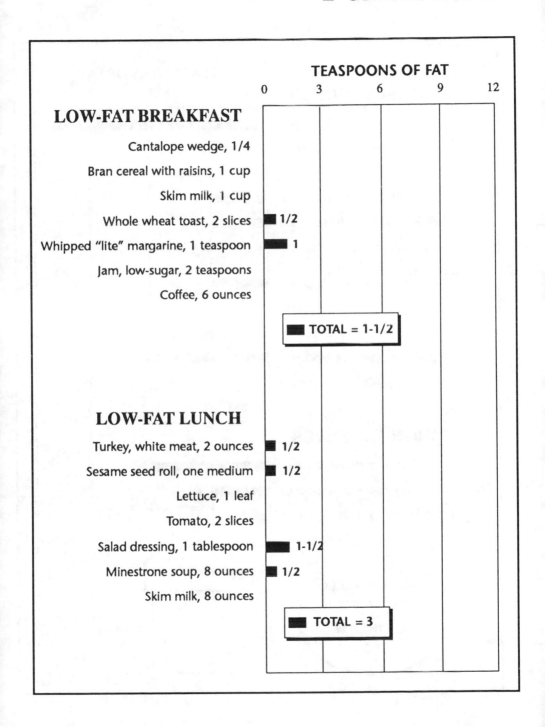

TEASPOONS OF FAT

0   3   6   9   12

LOW-FAT BREAKFAST

Cantalope wedge, 1/4

Bran cereal with raisins, 1 cup

Skim milk, 1 cup

Whole wheat toast, 2 slices — 1/2

Whipped "lite" margarine, 1 teaspoon — 1

Jam, low-sugar, 2 teaspoons

Coffee, 6 ounces

TOTAL = 1-1/2

LOW-FAT LUNCH

Turkey, white meat, 2 ounces — 1/2

Sesame seed roll, one medium — 1/2

Lettuce, 1 leaf

Tomato, 2 slices

Salad dressing, 1 tablespoon — 1-1/2

Minestrone soup, 8 ounces — 1/2

Skim milk, 8 ounces

TOTAL = 3

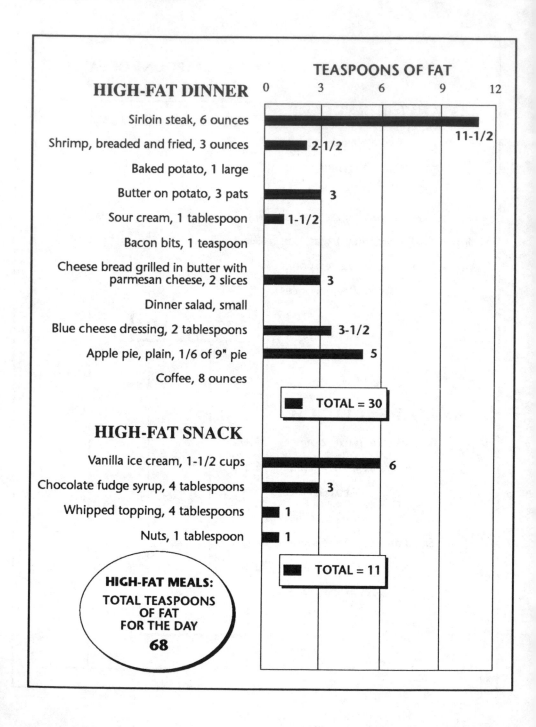

TEASPOONS OF FAT

HIGH-FAT DINNER

	Teaspoons of Fat
Sirloin steak, 6 ounces	11-1/2
Shrimp, breaded and fried, 3 ounces	2-1/2
Baked potato, 1 large	
Butter on potato, 3 pats	3
Sour cream, 1 tablespoon	1-1/2
Bacon bits, 1 teaspoon	
Cheese bread grilled in butter with parmesan cheese, 2 slices	3
Dinner salad, small	
Blue cheese dressing, 2 tablespoons	3-1/2
Apple pie, plain, 1/6 of 9" pie	5
Coffee, 8 ounces	

TOTAL = 30

HIGH-FAT SNACK

	Teaspoons of Fat
Vanilla ice cream, 1-1/2 cups	6
Chocolate fudge syrup, 4 tablespoons	3
Whipped topping, 4 tablespoons	1
Nuts, 1 tablespoon	1

TOTAL = 11

HIGH-FAT MEALS:
TOTAL TEASPOONS OF FAT FOR THE DAY
68

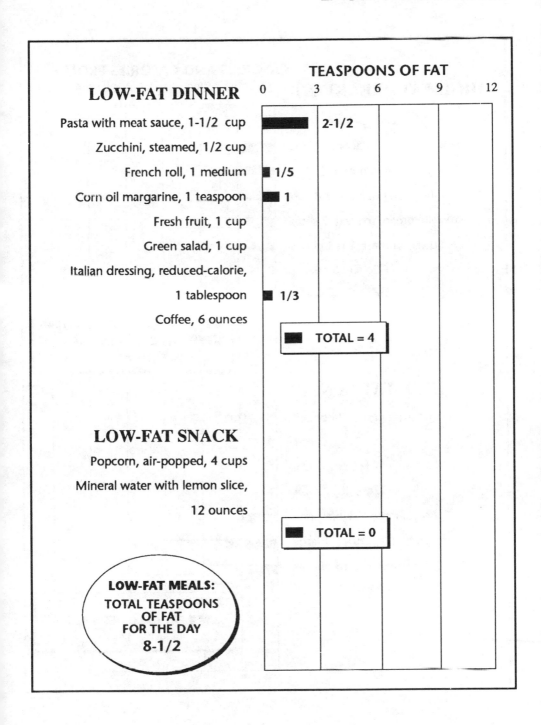

TEASPOONS OF FAT

LOW-FAT DINNER

0   3   6   9   12

Pasta with meat sauce, 1-1/2 cup   2-1/2

Zucchini, steamed, 1/2 cup

French roll, 1 medium   1/5

Corn oil margarine, 1 teaspoon   1

Fresh fruit, 1 cup

Green salad, 1 cup

Italian dressing, reduced-calorie,

1 tablespoon   1/3

Coffee, 6 ounces

TOTAL = 4

LOW-FAT SNACK

Popcorn, air-popped, 4 cups

Mineral water with lemon slice,

12 ounces

TOTAL = 0

LOW-FAT MEALS:
TOTAL TEASPOONS
OF FAT
FOR THE DAY
8-1/2

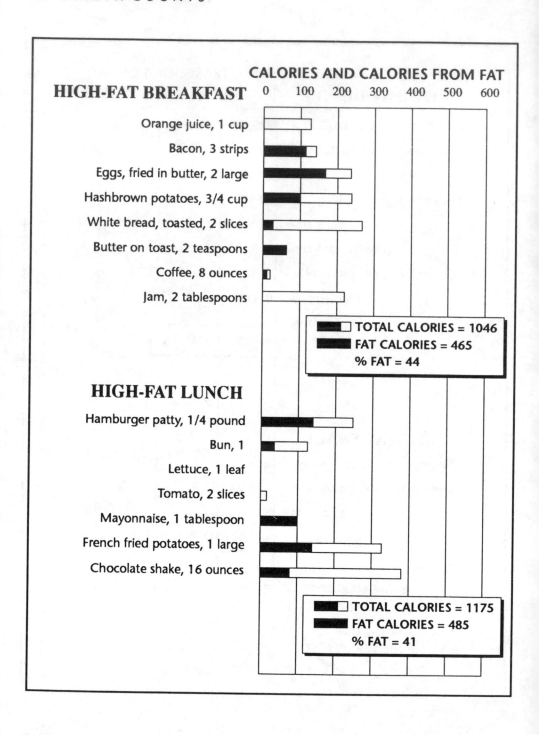

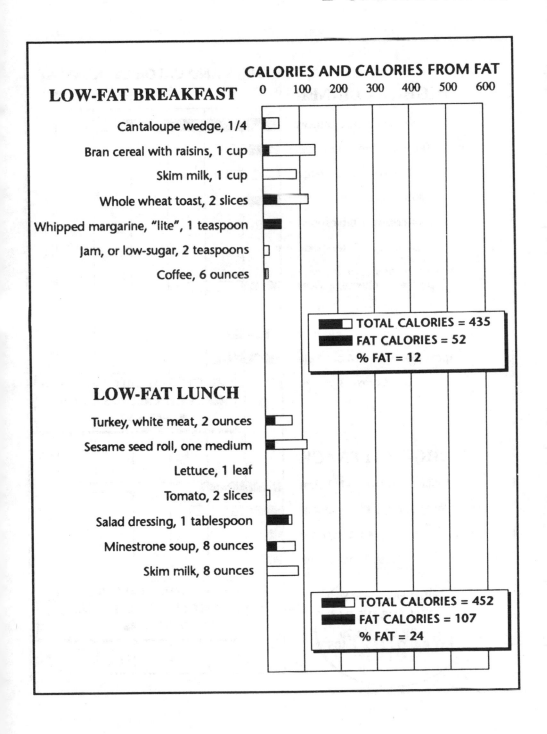

CALORIES AND CALORIES FROM FAT

LOW-FAT BREAKFAST

0   100   200   300   400   500   600

Cantaloupe wedge, 1/4

Bran cereal with raisins, 1 cup

Skim milk, 1 cup

Whole wheat toast, 2 slices

Whipped margarine, "lite", 1 teaspoon

Jam, or low-sugar, 2 teaspoons

Coffee, 6 ounces

TOTAL CALORIES = 435
FAT CALORIES = 52
% FAT = 12

LOW-FAT LUNCH

Turkey, white meat, 2 ounces

Sesame seed roll, one medium

Lettuce, 1 leaf

Tomato, 2 slices

Salad dressing, 1 tablespoon

Minestrone soup, 8 ounces

Skim milk, 8 ounces

TOTAL CALORIES = 452
FAT CALORIES = 107
% FAT = 24

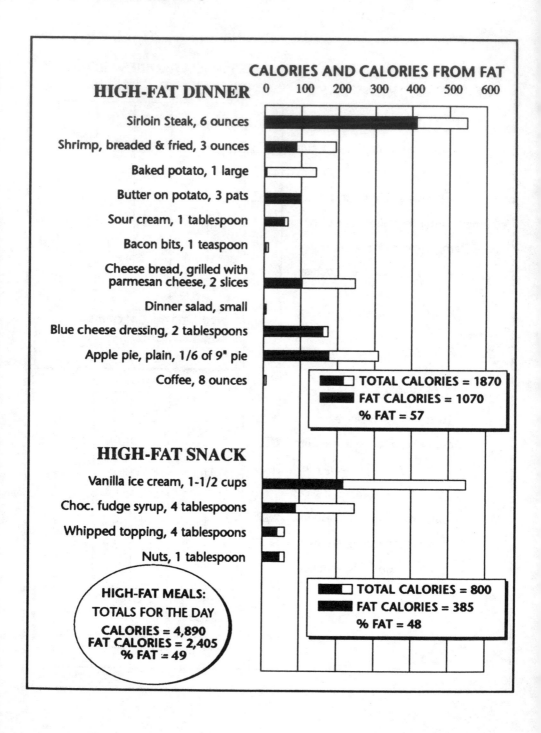

CALORIES AND CALORIES FROM FAT

HIGH-FAT DINNER

0   100   200   300   400   500   600

- Sirloin Steak, 6 ounces
- Shrimp, breaded & fried, 3 ounces
- Baked potato, 1 large
- Butter on potato, 3 pats
- Sour cream, 1 tablespoon
- Bacon bits, 1 teaspoon
- Cheese bread, grilled with parmesan cheese, 2 slices
- Dinner salad, small
- Blue cheese dressing, 2 tablespoons
- Apple pie, plain, 1/6 of 9" pie
- Coffee, 8 ounces

TOTAL CALORIES = 1870
FAT CALORIES = 1070
% FAT = 57

HIGH-FAT SNACK

- Vanilla ice cream, 1-1/2 cups
- Choc. fudge syrup, 4 tablespoons
- Whipped topping, 4 tablespoons
- Nuts, 1 tablespoon

TOTAL CALORIES = 800
FAT CALORIES = 385
% FAT = 48

HIGH-FAT MEALS:
TOTALS FOR THE DAY
CALORIES = 4,890
FAT CALORIES = 2,405
% FAT = 49

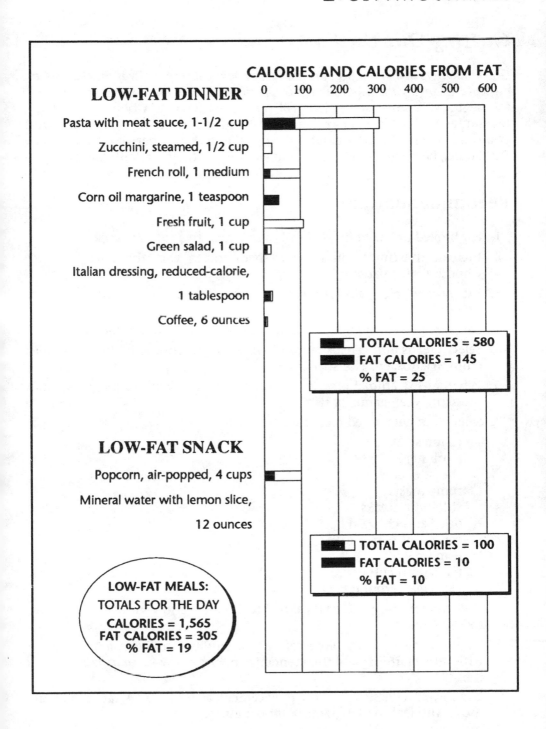

CALORIES AND CALORIES FROM FAT

LOW-FAT DINNER

0   100   200   300   400   500   600

Pasta with meat sauce, 1-1/2 cup

Zucchini, steamed, 1/2 cup

French roll, 1 medium

Corn oil margarine, 1 teaspoon

Fresh fruit, 1 cup

Green salad, 1 cup

Italian dressing, reduced-calorie,

1 tablespoon

Coffee, 6 ounces

TOTAL CALORIES = 580
FAT CALORIES = 145
% FAT = 25

LOW-FAT SNACK

Popcorn, air-popped, 4 cups

Mineral water with lemon slice,

12 ounces

TOTAL CALORIES = 100
FAT CALORIES = 10
% FAT = 10

LOW-FAT MEALS:
TOTALS FOR THE DAY
CALORIES = 1,565
FAT CALORIES = 305
% FAT = 19

Cutting Out the Fat

Good managers realize changes are not made overnight. Especially if the changes are difficult. Changing the way you eat takes patience, humor and determination.

Begin with small steps that will make a difference. Choose one of the recommendations listed below and start to cut out fat today. When you find you can easily fit this new habit into your life, pick another. *And then another.* Remember, begin with the easiest and work up to the more difficult changes.

Recommendations

1. Eat broiled or baked fish instead of red meat two times a week.
2. Increase the times you select fresh or frozen vegetables over canned. Choose a wide variety.
3. Eat more whole grains and cereals. They add bulk, not calories, and are rich in fiber and nutrients.
4. Eat *plant* protein such as beans and breads in place of red meat.
5. Select breads and cereals more often than you choose high-fat crackers, chips, nachos, etc., for snacks.
6. When eating animal protein, choose low-fat chicken or turkey (without the skin), veal, game, or fish.
7. Select lean cuts of red meat such as:
   round steak
   flank steak
   shoulder cuts
   rump roasts
   sirloin tip steaks
   dried and chipped beef
   center cut ham steaks
   lean stew meat
   tenderloin cuts
   extra-lean ground beef
8. Keep your portions of red meat to 3 to 4 ounces and your fish and poultry to 3 to 6 ounces.
9. Examine meat for marbling before you buy it. *Marbling is fat.* Pick a cut with little marbling and then tenderize it with a low-fat marinade or cook it in the crock pot.
10. Use low-fat cheese as a meat replacement at meals. Low-fat cheeses are those with less than 4 grams of fat per ounce.

11. Avoid using cheese for snacks. In just a few bites you can load on the calories and fat.

12. Replace high-fat lunch meats such as bologna, braunsweiger, bacon, sausage, or hotdogs with lower-fat varieties. Select luncheon meats with no more than 2–3 grams of fat per ounce.

    For example, choose turkey hotdogs, turkey pastrami, turkey ham, smoked turkey breast, lean ham, etc. If it's at least 95% lean, it's a good choice.

13. Select low-fat or skim milk dairy products: milk, cheese, yogurt, and cottage cheese.

14. When eating high-fat desserts and pastries, eat a smaller portion.

15. Plan your high-fat eating (snack, dessert, candy) and *make it a special event during the week rather than often each day.*

16. Buy a new low-fat cookbook. Read the introduction and try out some of the recipes.

17. Swap a good low-fat recipe with a friend and try it out next week.

Techniques

1. Trim all visible fat from animal protein, including the skin from poultry, before cooking.

2. Broil, boil, roast, stew, barbecue, microwave or bake meats, fish and poultry instead of frying.

3. Skim the fat off broths and soups. Prepare them in advance and refrigerate then so that the fat hardens on top.

4. Use recipes that have little or no added fat. You can also reduce fat by 1/3 to 1/2 in most recipes without losing flavor and texture. Experiment!

5. Cut the fat in half when cooking or baking. Most cookbooks and family recipes were written before we realized that a diet high in fat is unhealthy.

6. Cut in half—or eliminate—the margarine, butter, mayonnaise, cream cheese, salad dressing, and sauces you usually put on foods.

7. Substitute cocoa powder for chocolate bars in cooking. Three tablespoons of cocoa equals 1 square ounce of chocolate.

8. To brown meat, use a non-stick pan and add no fat.

9. To stir-fry, use water rather than oil.

Tracking Calories and Calories from Fat

Now your work as a fat detective begins in earnest. Use your food diary to write down everything you eat or drink during the day. Then add these new steps.

1. Review "Keeping a Food Diary." The directions and sample will help you learn how to fill in the total calories and calories from fat columns in your food diary.

2. Look up each food and drink item.

3. Calculate the total calories and calories from fat for the size portion you ate.

4. Also note the percentage fat column for that food item. Is it high or low? If it is greater than 30%, take a highlight pen and highlight that food entry in your food diary. At the end of the day you can see at a glance what foods are high in fat and how many high-fat foods you chose that day.

5. At the end of the day, add the total calories column and the calories from fat column. Then calculate the percentage of calories from fat for the entire day.

$$\frac{\text{TOTAL CALORIES FROM FAT}}{\text{TOTAL CALORIES}} = \text{PERCENTAGE CALORIES FROM FAT}$$

6. When you finish your calculations, take a few minutes to study your diary.

   - What foods are highest in calories? Are they also high in fat?
   - Were they worth it? Could you somehow lower the percentage of fat in them without giving up the foods? How?
     See the "Cooking Tips: Cutting Down on Fat" section on pages 16–17 and the "Cutting Out the Fat" guidelines in this chapter for practical suggestions.
   - Do you want to substitute something less fattening? How can you plan for that tomorrow?
   - What is your percentage of calories from fat for the day? If you take out the two foods that are highest in fat and recalculate your percentage of calories from fat for the day, how much does it drop? Look good?

Your work as a detective is cut out for you.

- Find the high-fat foods.
- Cut back on the fat or reduce the serving size.
- Or—cut the fat foods altogether and substitute a food that tastes just as good, helps you build a healthier body—and doesn't leave any tell-tale traces around your middle!

Keeping track of calories and percentage of calories from fat puts you back in charge of your eating.

- You collect the information you need to decide what changes you must make.
- You explore choices and options.
- You pick solutions that you judge will work best for you.
- You try them out and make adjustments.

You are becoming a skillful planner and decision-maker. You are gaining wisdom and losing weight. You are in charge.

Use the next two pages to develop your own quick-reference list of the foods you eat most often.

FOOD		CALORIES		
	AMOUNT	TOTAL	FAT	%FAT

FOOD		CALORIES		
	AMOUNT	TOTAL	FAT	%FAT

APHABETICAL FOOD LIST

FOOD

CALORIES

	AMOUNT	TOTAL	FAT	%FAT

A

	AMOUNT	TOTAL	FAT	%FAT
Abalone, raw	1 oz	30	2	6
Acorn squash, baked, 1/2 squash	1/2 cup	65	9	14
Ale	12 oz	147	0	0
Alfalfa sprouts	1/2 cup	12	1	8
All Bran (Kellogg's)	1 cup	210	27	13
Almond bark, white dipping chocolate	1 oz	82	14	17
Almond cookie, Chinese, 2" diameter	1 cookie	153	97	63
Almond Delight (Ralston)	1 cup	147	11	7
Almond Joy, 1.76oz	1 bar	250	126	50
Almond Roca	1 oz	164	99	60
Almonds, whole				
22 = 1 oz	1 oz	153	137	90
5 oz = 1 cup	1 cup	765	684	89
American cheese, processed				
(Velveeta)	1 oz	80	54	68
reduced fat (Kraft)	1 oz	70	36	51
slice	1 oz	95	62	65
American cheese spread, processed	1 oz	80	53	66
Anchovies				
canned in oil	1 oz	60	25	42
pickled	1 oz	49	26	53
Angel food cake, mix, tube, 9 3/4"				
1/12 of mix	1 piece	135	tr	tr
whole cake	1 cake	1620	1	tr
Animal crackers	5 crackers	43	8	19

Abbreviations and symbols:

lb = pound	oz = ounce	Tbsp = Tablespoon
tsp = teaspoon	tr = trace	pkg = package

✔ = homemade, a standard cookbook recipe we have not changed to lower fat. Use the check to remind yourself *you can modify recipes*. See page 16 for tips on lowering fat in any recipe without losing quality or flavor.

FOOD

CALORIES

	AMOUNT	TOTAL	FAT	%FAT
Antipasto, raw vegetable ✔	1 cup	355	297	84
Apple, fresh, 3" diameter	1 apple	96	8	8
dried	1 oz	83	8	10
1.4 oz = 1/2 cup	1/2 cup	117	6	5
Apple brown betty ✔	1/2 cup	211	44	21
Apple butter	1 Tbsp	33	1	3
Apple chips	1 oz	120	45	38
Apple cobbler ✔	3/4 cup	505	198	39
Apple crisp ✔	1/2 cup	302	73	24
Apple dumplings ✔	1 cup	755	297	39
Apple fritters (Mrs. Paul's)	1 piece	120	53	44
Apple Jacks (Kellogg's)	1 cup	110	0	0
Apple juice				
canned or frozen, reconstituted,				
unsweetened	8 oz	120	tr	tr
frozen, concentrate	6 oz	270	tr	tr
Apple pie				
(Burger King)	1 serving	305	108	35
(McDonald's)	1 serving	260	133	51
Apple pie, double crust ✔				
1/6 of 9"	1 piece	403	174	43
1/8 of 9"	1 piece	302	131	43
9", whole	1 pie	2416	1044	43
Apple pie, snack size (Sara Lee)	1 pie	230	81	35
Apple spice muffin (Dunkin' Donuts)	1 muffin	327	99	30
Apple strudel, frozen (Pepperidge Farm)	1 serving	290	129	44
Apple turnover, 3 oz ✔	1 turnover	255	127	50
Apple-raisin muffins ✔	1 muffin	201	81	40
Applesauce coffee cake ✔	1/8 cake	307	144	47
Applesauce spice cake, 3 x 3 x 1" ✔	1 piece	136	90	66
Applesauce, canned				
sweetened	1/2 cup	115	tr	tr
unsweetened	1/2 cup	50	tr	tr
Apricots, dried				
4 halves	1 oz	74	1	1
2.7 oz = 1/2 cup	1/2 cup	200	3	2

FOOD

CALORIES

	AMOUNT	TOTAL	FAT	%FAT
Apricots				
canned				
heavy syrup	1/2 cup	110	tr	tr
juice pack	1/2 cup	54	2	4
water pack	1/2 cup	38	1	3
fresh, whole	3 apricots	55	2	4
Apricot nectar, canned	8 oz	145	tr	tr
Arrowroot	1 Tbsp	30	0	0
Arrowroot cookie (Nabisco)	1 cookie	23	7	30
Arroz con pollo, with 1/2 cup rice ✔	4 oz meat	403	90	22
Artichoke hearts, frozen	1/2 cup	20	tr	tr
Artichokes with butter sauce ✔	1 average	232	207	89
Artichokes				
medium	1 medium	53	2	4
Jerusalem, small, 1 1/2" diameter	1 small	17	tr	tr
Asparagus				
canned, cut	1/2 cup	22	3	14
fresh or canned, spears, 1/2" diameter	4 spears	15	tr	tr
Avacado dressing ✔	1 Tbsp	34	27	79
Avocado				
cubed	1/2 cup	125	110	88
mashed	1/2 cup	276	243	88
whole, peeled, 4" diameter	1 average	378	333	88

B

	AMOUNT	TOTAL	FAT	%FAT
Babka, 8" diameter	1 roll	1361	926	68
Bac-O-Bits (General Mills)	1 Tbsp	38	14	37

FOOD

CALORIES

	AMOUNT	TOTAL	FAT	%FAT
Bacon				
broiled or fried, crisp	2 slices	85	72	85
Canadian	1 oz	61	37	61
Imitation Crumbles (R.T. French)	1 tsp	6	tr	tr
Bacon, lettuce, tomato sandwich on white	1 sandwich	352	197	56
Bacon Swiss burger (Wendy's)	1 burger	710	396	56
Baileys Irish Cream	1 oz	118	25	21
Bagel sandwich, breakfast (Burger King)	1 sandwich	387	126	33
Bagel with egg, 3 1/2" diameter, plain	1 bagel	180	13	7
Bagel without egg, 3 1/2" diameter				
garlic	1 bagel	180	9	5
onion	1 bagel	180	9	5
plain	1 bagel	170	9	5
raisin honey	1 bagel	180	9	5
Baked Alaska, 1/8 of 9 x 9 x 2" ✔	1 serving	557	21	4
Baked beans, canned				
with pork, tomato sauce	1/2 cup	156	30	19
with sweet sauce	1/2 cup	191	54	28
vegetarian, without pork	1/2 cup	153	6	4
Baked potato				
plain, 5 x 2 ", medium	1 potato	145	2	1
plain, large (Wendy's)	1 potato	250	18	7
with cheese, bacon (Wendy's)	1 potato	570	270	47
with sour cream, chives (Wendy's)	1 potato	460	216	47
Baklava, walnut, 1 x 2"	1 piece	117	55	47
Bamboo shoots				
canned	1/2 cup	11	tr	tr
fresh	1/2 cup	18	2	11
Banana bread				
5 x 4 1/2 x 1/2"	1/18 loaf	136	52	38
9 x 5 x 4 1/2" loaf	1 loaf	2441	941	39
Banana chips, dehydrated	1 oz	103	10	10
Banana cream pie				
1/6 of 9"	1 piece	413	168	41
1/8 of 9"	1 piece	309	126	41
9", whole	1 pie	2478	1008	41

FOOD | CALORIES

	AMOUNT	TOTAL	FAT	%FAT
Banana flakes	1 Tbsp	20	tr	tr
Banana nut bread ✔	1/16 loaf	154	54	35
Banana nut muffin (Dunkin' Donuts)	1 muffin	327	108	33
Banana split (Dairy Queen)	1 serving	540	99	18
Banana, medium, 7"	1 banana	100	2	2
Barbecue sauce	1 Tbsp	20	4	20
	1/2 cup	160	32	20
Barbeque spareribs, meat only	1 oz	145	107	74
Barbeque pork, without bone	1 oz	54	32	59
Barley, pearled, pot or Scotch				
cooked	1 cup	199	5	3
dry	1 cup	698	2	tr
Bass, Sea, broiled	1 oz	35	6	17
Bean dip, canned (Frito Lay)	1/4 cup	66	25	38
Bean sprouts, mung, raw or cooked	1/2 cup	18	tr	tr
Bean threads, cooked	1 cup	98	tr	tr
Bean with bacon soup (Campbell's)	1 cup	145	32	22
Bean with pork soup, with water	1 cup	170	54	32
Beans, green, cut, fresh cooked,				
canned or frozen	1/2 cup	15	tr	tr
Beans, refried, plain or spicy	1 cup	248	16	6
Beans, yellow, cut, fresh cooked,				
canned or frozen	1/2 cup	18	tr	tr
Beef (Land O'Frost)	1 oz	40	18	45
Beef 'n cheddar sandwich (Arby's)	1 sandwich	455	241	53
Beef and vegetable stir-fry, with rice ✔	1 1/2 cups	513	189	37
Beef broth				
condensed (Campbell's)	1 cup	46	0	0
reconstituted, with water (Campbell's)	1 cup	23	0	0
Beef Fajitas, frozen (Weight Watchers)	6 3/4 oz	260	54	21
Beef jerky	1 oz	108	43	40
Beef kebabs ✔	1 kebab	358	207	58
Beef noodle soup	1 cup	65	27	42
Beef Pepper Steak, frozen (Tyson)	11 1/4 oz	330	99	30
Beef potpie, 4 1/4" diameter ✔	1 pie	558	296	53

FOOD

CALORIES

	AMOUNT	TOTAL	FAT	%FAT
Beef stew				
canned (Nalley)	1 cup	190	54	28
homemade ✔	1 cup	225	77	34
Beef Stroganoff, frozen (Armour)	10 oz	320	108	34
Beef stroganoff, with noodles ✔	1 1/2 cups	735	495	67
Beef teriyaki ✔	4 oz beef	429	315	73
Beef tongue, simmered	1 oz	80	53	66
Beef with pea pods, Chinese	1 cup	321	203	63
Beef, brisket, braised	1 oz	68	33	49
Beef, chuck, arm pot roast, braised	1 oz	65	25	38
Beef, dried	1 oz	47	10	21
Beef, eye of round, roasted	1 oz	52	17	33
Beef, ground				
extra lean, 15% fat				
1 lb raw = 12 oz cooked	12 oz	804	444	55
baked	1 oz	67	36	54
broiled	1 oz	68	37	54
pan-fried	1 oz	67	37	55
lean, 20% fat				
1 lb raw = 11 1/2 oz cooked	11 1/2 oz	886	541	61
baked	1 oz	75	45	60
broiled	1 oz	76	46	60
pan-fried	1 oz	77	47	61
regular, 27% fat				
1 lb raw = 11 oz cooked	11 oz	957	649	68
baked	1 oz	82	54	66
broiled	1 oz	83	54	65
pan-fried	1 oz	87	59	68
Beef, heart, simmered	1 oz	49	14	29
Beef, liver, fried	1 oz	65	27	42
Beef, rib, large end, roasted	1 oz	69	36	52
small end, roasted	1 oz	62	29	47
Beef, short ribs, braised	1 oz	84	46	55
Beef, top round, broiled	1 oz	54	16	30
Beef-barley soup ✔	1 cup	343	189	55
Beefaroni (Chef Boyardee)	1 cup	213	54	25

FOOD | CALORIES

	AMOUNT	TOTAL	FAT	%FAT
Beer, light				
Bud Light (Budweiser)	12 oz	108	0	0
Lite (Miller)	12 oz	96	0	0
Oly Gold (Olympia)	12 oz	70	0	0
Beer, regular	12 oz	168	0	0
Beet greens, cooked, leaves and stems	1/2 cup	13	tr	tr
Beets				
canned, pickled	1/2 cup	81	tr	tr
canned, whole baby	1/2 cup	36	tr	tr
fresh cooked, canned, sliced or diced	1/2 cup	30	tr	tr
Better Cheddars (Nabisco)	1 cracker	6	3	50
Big Classic burger (Wendy's)	1 burger	580	306	53
with cheese	1 burger	640	360	56
Big Country breakfast with ham (Hardee's)	1 serving	620	297	48
Big Mac hamburger (McDonald's)	1 burger	560	292	52
Big Twin burger (Hardee's)	1 burger	450	225	50
Biscuit (Dunkin' Donuts)	1 biscuit	332	207	62
Biscuit (Hardee's)				
bacon, egg, and cheese	1 biscuit	460	252	55
Canadian Rise 'N Shine	1 biscuit	470	243	52
chicken	1 biscuit	430	198	46
sausage	1 biscuit	440	252	57
sausage and egg	1 biscuit	490	279	57
steak	1 biscuit	500	261	52
Biscuit (McDonald's)				
with bacon, egg and cheese	1 biscuit	440	238	54
with sausage	1 biscuit	440	261	59
with sausage and egg	1 biscuit	520	311	60
with spread	1 bisucit	260	114	44
Biscuits				
buttermilk	1 biscuit	82	37	45
2" diameter	1 biscuit	105	45	43
refrigerator (Pillsbury)	1 biscuit	100	36	36
BK Broiler chicken sandwich (Burger King)	1 sandwich	379	162	43
Black bean soup (Campbell's)	1 cup	110	18	16

FOOD	AMOUNT	CALORIES		
		TOTAL	FAT	%FAT
Black beans, cooked	1 cup	280	12	4
dry	1 cup	678	28	4
Black bottom pie ✔				
1/6 of 9"	1 piece	576	252	44
1/8 of 9"	1 piece	432	189	44
9", whole	1 pie	3456	1512	44
Black Forest cake, 1/12, with frosting ✔	1 piece	661	31	5
Blackberries, fresh	1/2 cup	43	4	9
Blackberry pie, double crust ✔				
1/6 of 9"	1 piece	383	156	41
1/8 of 9"	1 piece	287	117	41
9", whole	1 pie	2296	936	41
Blackeyed peas, cowpeas, cooked	1 cup	178	12	7
raw	1 cup	184	10	5
Blintz, cheese, fruit filled, 6"	1 blintz	164	33	20
Blizzard, 16 oz (Dairy Queen)				
Butterfinger	1 serving	765	252	33
Hawaiian	1 serving	700	198	28
Heath	1 serving	800	216	27
Strawberry	1 serving	675	153	23
Bloody Mary	6 oz	160	0	0
Blue cheese	1 oz	103	77	75
Blue cheese salad dressing				
reduced calorie	1 Tbsp	11	7	64
regular	1 Tbsp	71	66	93
(Burger King)	1 packet	300	279	93
(McDonald's)	1 packet	350	311	89
Blueberries, fresh	1/2 cup	45	4	9
Blueberry muffin, 3" diameter	1 muffin	298	171	58
4" diameter	1 muffin	397	229	58
(Dunkin' Donuts)	1 muffin	263	90	34
Blueberry pancake, 4" diameter	1 pancake	134	27	20
Blueberry pie, double crust				
1/6 of 9"	1 piece	381	153	40
1/8 of 9"	1 piece	286	114	40
9", whole	1 pie	2287	919	40

FOOD

CALORIES

	AMOUNT	TOTAL	FAT	%FAT
Bluefish, broiled or baked	1 oz	44	13	30
Bockwurst	1 oz	74	59	80
Bologna	1 oz	88	73	83
Boston brown bread, canned, 3 1/4 x 1/2"	1 slice	95	8	8
Boston cream pie ✔				
1/6 of 8"	1 piece	415	114	27
1/8 of 8"	1 piece	311	86	28
8", whole	1 pie	2490	686	28
Bouillabaisse ✔	1 cup	245	84	34
Bouillon cube, dehydrated	1 cube	5	tr	tr
Bowties, pasta, cooked	1 cup	100	9	9
dry	1 cup	200	18	9
Boysenberries, fresh, canned or				
frozen, unsweetened	1/2 cup	44	1	2
Bran Buds (Kellogg's)	1 cup	210	27	13
Bran cereal with raisins	1 cup	145	9	6
Bran Checks (Ralston)	1 cup	165	12	7
Bran Flakes, 40%	1 cup	105	9	9
Bran muffin				
with raisins, 3" diameter	1 muffin	271	58	21
4" diameter	1 muffin	361	77	21
(Dunkin' Donuts)	1 muffin	353	117	33
from mix (Duncan Hines)	1 muffin	100	27	27
Bran, oat	1 Tbsp	21	3	14
	1 cup	330	54	16
Bran, wheat, unprocessed or miller's	1 Tbsp	7	tr	tr
	1 cup	111	22	20
Brandy	1 oz	73	0	0
Brandy Alexander, with 3 Tbsp cream	3 oz	237	100	42
Branola bread, 5 x 3 1/2 x 1/2"	1 slice	100	9	9
Braunschweiger	1 oz	102	82	80
Brazil nuts, whole				
3 = 1 oz	1 oz	173	159	92
5.3 oz = 1 cup	1 cup	916	840	92
Bread and butter pickles ✔	1/4 cup	95	0	0

FOOD	AMOUNT	CALORIES		
		TOTAL	FAT	%FAT
Bread crumbs				
dry, grated	1 cup	346	36	10
white, fresh	1 cup	120	9	8
Bread pudding with raisins ✔	1/2 cup	209	60	29
Bread sticks, hard, 7x1/2"	1 stick	27	2	7
Bread				
rye, 4 3/4 x 3 3/4 x 7/16"	1 slice	60	tr	tr
white, 4 1/2 x 4 x 1/2"	1 slice	70	9	13
sandwich, 4 x 4 x 1/2"	1 slice	60	9	15
whole wheat, 4 1/2 x 4 x 1/2"	1 slice	60	9	15
sandwich, 4 x 4 x 1/2"	1 slice	45	9	20
whole wheat, 100% stone ground, 5 x 4 1/2 x 1/2"	1 slice	100	9	9
Bread, Light (Wonder)				
Oatmeal, 4 x 4 x 1/2"	1 slice	40	4	10
Sourdough, 4 x 4 x 3/4"	1 slice	40	4	10
Wheat, 3 1/2 x 4 x 1/2"	1 slice	40	4	10
Bread, toasted				
white, 4 1/2 x 4 x 1/2"	1 slice	70	9	13
whole wheat, 4 1/2 x 4 x 1/2"	1 slice	60	9	15
Breakfast sandwich (Wendy's)	1 sandwich	370	171	46
Brick cheese	1 oz	105	72	69
Brie cheese	1 oz	95	71	75
Broccoli				
fresh cooked or frozen				
chopped	1/2 cup	25	tr	tr
stalk	1 average	40	tr	tr
raw				
chopped	1/2 cup	12	tr	tr
stalk	1 average	42	tr	tr
Broccoli and cheese sauce, frozen	1/2 cup	70	18	26
Brotwurst	1 oz	90	72	80
Brown sugar, packed	1/2 cup	410	0	0
	1 Tbsp	51	0	0
	1 tsp	17	0	0

FOOD		CALORIES		
	AMOUNT	TOTAL	FAT	%FAT
Brownie				
chocolate, plain, 2" square ✔	1 brownie	146	85	58
(Dunkin' Donuts)	1 brownie	280	117	42
fudge, 1/24 mix (Betty Crocker)	1 brownie	130	45	35
	1 mix	3120	1080	35
with walnuts, 1/24 mix				
(Betty Crocker)	1 brownie	160	63	39
	1 mix	3840	1512	39
Brussels sprouts and butter sauce, frozen	1/2 cup	60	9	15
Brussels sprouts, fresh or frozen, cooked	1/2 cup	28	4	14
Buckwheat pancakes				
4" diameter	1 pancake	108	46	43
6" diameter	1 pancake	146	59	40
Bulgur, cooked	1 cup	226	9	4
dry	1 cup	600	23	4
Bun, hamburger or frankfurter	1 bun	110	18	16
Burrito				
bean (Taco Bell)	1 burrito	357	92	26
bean and cheese, 5 oz	1 burrito	339	99	29
beef (Taco Bell)	1 burrito	403	156	39
beef and bean, 5 oz	1 burrito	366	135	37
double beef supreme (Taco Bell)	1 burrito	457	196	43
green chili, 5 oz	1 burrito	353	117	33
red hot beef, 5 oz	1 burrito	319	109	34
supreme (Taco Bell)	1 burrito	413	158	38
Buster bar (Dairy Queen)	1 serving	460	261	57
Butter Buds, reconstituted	1 Tbsp	6	0	0
	1 oz	12	0	0
Butter cookie, spritz	1 cookie	23	8	35
Butter, regular	1 tsp	34	34	100
	1 pat	36	36	100
	1 Tbsp	102	102	100
	1 cup	1625	1625	100
Butter, whipped	1 tsp	23	23	100
	1 Tbsp	67	67	100
	1 cup	1081	1081	100

FOOD

CALORIES

	AMOUNT	TOTAL	FAT	%FAT
Buttermilk biscuit	1 biscuit	82	37	45
(Kentucky Fried Chicken)	1 biscuit	232	107	46
(Wendy's)	1 biscuit	320	153	48
Buttermilk creamy dressing	1 Tbsp	80	72	90
Buttermilk dressing ✔	1 Tbsp	41	32	78
Buttermilk oat bran bread, 4 x 5 x 1/2"	1 slice	80	18	23
Buttermilk pancake				
4" diameter	1 pancake	110	28	25
5" diameter (Krusteaz)	1 pancake	103	15	15
Buttermilk waffle mix, dry (Aunt Jemima)	1 cup	510	27	5
Buttermilk waffles, frozen	1 medium	90	24	27
Buttermilk				
cultured, powder, reconstituted	1 cup	79	6	8
dried	1/2 cup	233	31	13
skim	1 cup	88	2	2
Butterscotch candy, hard	1 piece	20	2	10
Butterscotch caramel topping (Smucker's)	1 Tbsp	45	tr	tr
Butterscotch chips, 3 oz = 1/2 cup	1/2 cup	456	237	52
60 pieces = 1 oz	1 oz	152	79	52

C

	AMOUNT	TOTAL	FAT	%FAT
Cabbage rolls, stuffed with ground beef	1 medium	193	95	49
Cabbage				
Chinese, raw	1/2 cup	6	tr	tr
cooked	1/2 cup	12	tr	tr
green or red, chopped or shredded	1/2 cup	10	tr	tr
green or red, cooked, drained	1/2 cup	15	tr	tr
Savoy, raw, chopped	1/2 cup	8	tr	tr

FOOD | CALORIES

	AMOUNT	TOTAL	FAT	%FAT
Caesar salad dressing	1 Tbsp	70	63	90
(McDonald's)	1 packet	300	275	92
Calf liver				
fried	1 oz	75	34	45
raw	1 oz	40	12	30
Camembert cheese	1 oz	84	62	74
Candied fruit				
cherry, for baking	1 cherry	12	tr	tr
citron, for fruit cake	1 oz	89	1	1
pineapple slice	1 slice	120	2	2
Candied squash ✔	1/2 squash	164	36	22
Candy, hard, 1/4 oz	1 piece	25	0	0
sugar free	1 piece	25	0	0
Cannelloni ✔	1 each	134	45	34
Cantaloupe, fresh, 5" diameter	1/2 melon	82	3	4
cubed	1/2 cup	24	2	8
Caramels, plain or chocolate (Kraft)	1 piece	35	9	26
Caraway cheese	1 oz	107	75	70
Cardamom bread ✔	1 piece	89	27	30
Carmel apples ✔	1 apple	427	90	21
Carmel corn ✔	1 cup	199	81	41
Carob covered almonds	1 oz	150	108	72
Carob drops/stars	1 oz	116	14	12
Carrot cake				
1/12, without frosting (Betty Crocker)	1 piece	260	108	42
with cream cheese frosting, 2" square	1 piece	334	157	47
without frosting (Betty Crocker)	1 cake	3120	1296	42
Carrot salad				
with nuts, raisins, sour cream	1/2 cup	383	189	49
with raisins and mayonnaise	1/2 cup	141	66	47
Carrots				
raw, 7 1/2"	1 carrot	30	tr	tr
fresh cooked, canned, sliced, drained	1/2 cup	23	tr	tr
raw, grated	1/2 cup	23	tr	tr
Casaba melon, fresh,				
6 1/2" diameter, 2" wedge	1 wedge	38	tr	tr

FOOD

CALORIES

	AMOUNT	TOTAL	FAT	%FAT
Cashews				
18 = 1 oz	1 oz	161	115	71
5 oz = 1 cup	1 cup	805	575	71
Catalina salad dressing, reduced calorie	1 Tbsp	16	0	0
Catsup	1/2 cup	145	4	3
	1 Tbsp	15	tr	tr
Cauliflower				
fresh or frozen, cooked	1/2 cup	15	tr	tr
raw, chopped	1/2 cup	16	tr	tr
with cheese sauce, frozen	5 oz	130	63	48
Caviar, Sturgeon	1 Tbsp	42	22	52
Celery				
diced	1/2 cup	10	tr	tr
large stalk	1 stalk	5	tr	tr
Cereal party mix	1 cup	418	261	62
Champagne	4 oz	84	0	0
Chayotte, squash, raw	1 medium	56	2	4
Cheddar cheese food spread				
sharp (Kraft)	1 oz	90	63	70
with wine (Kraft)	1 oz	90	54	60
Cheddar cheese	1 oz	112	82	73
grated or shredded	1/2 cup	229	167	73
Light Natural (Kraft)	1 oz	80	45	56
Cheddar macaroni salad ✔	1/2 cup	196	117	60
Chee-tos, cheese flavor snack, 57 = 1 3/4 oz	1 3/4 oz	280	153	55
Cheerios, regular or Apple Cinnamon				
(General Mills)	1 cup	88	14	16
Cheese ball ✔	1 Tbsp	64	54	84
Cheese bread ✔	1/16 loaf	70	18	26
Cheese dog (Dairy Queen)	1 serving	330	189	57
Cheese fondue ✔	1/4 cup	170	105	62
Cheese, low-fat (Olympia)	1 oz	87	54	62
Cheese omelet ✔	2 eggs	379	288	76
Cheese Pizza, frozen (Banquet Kid Cuisine)	6.5 oz	240	36	15
Cheese puffs, snack food, 25 = 1 cup	1 cup	96	54	56

FOOD	AMOUNT	CALORIES		
		TOTAL	FAT	%FAT
Cheese sauce ✔	1/4 cup	132	88	67
	1 Tbsp	33	22	67
Cheese spread, processed (Cheez Whiz)	1 oz	80	54	68
Cheeseburger				
(McDonald's)	1 burger	310	124	40
bacon, double (Burger King)	1 burger	510	279	55
deluxe (Burger King)	1 burger	364	180	49
regular (Burger King)	1 burger	317	135	43
double (Dairy Queen)	1 burger	650	333	51
single (Dairy Queen)	1 burger	410	180	44
triple (Dairy Queen)	1 burger	820	450	55
plain, 1/4 pound (Wendy's)	1 burger	410	198	48
single with everything (Wendy's)	1 burger	490	252	51
small (Wendy's)	1 burger	320	135	42
Cheesecake ✔				
Classic, snack size (Sara Lee)	1 cake	200	126	63
1/8 of 8" diameter	1 piece	414	251	61
8" diameter	1 cake	3312	2008	61
with cherry sauce	1/12 cake	482	261	54
Cheez-It (Sunshine)	1 cracker	6	3	50
Cheezola	1 oz	90	63	70
Chef salad, with 2 Tbsp dressing	2 1/2 cups	480	302	63
Chef salad, without dressing	2 1/2 cups	320	162	51
(Burger King)	1 salad	180	81	45
(Hardee's)	1 salad	240	135	56
(McDonald's)	1 salad	230	120	52
(Wendy's)	1 salad	180	81	45
Cherimoya	1 average	515	20	4
Cherries				
canned				
sour/red, water pack	1/2 cup	53	tr	tr
in heavy syrup	1/2 cup	116	tr	tr
sweet, water pack	1/2 cup	43	2	5
juice pack	1/2 cup	68	tr	tr
fresh	10 cherries	45	tr	tr
Maraschino, large	1 cherry	10	0	0

FOOD

CALORIES

	AMOUNT	TOTAL	FAT	%FAT
Cherry muffin (Dunkin' Donuts)	1 muffin	317	90	28
Cherry pie, double crust ✔				
1/6 of 9"	1 piece	411	160	39
1/8 of 9"	1 piece	308	120	39
9", whole	1 pie	2466	961	39
Cheshire cheese	1 oz	110	77	70
Chestnuts, fresh, 4 large or 6 small	1 oz	58	4	7
Chicken a L' Orange, frozen (Lean Cuisine)	8 oz	260	54	21
Chicken 'a la king ✔	1 cup	233	121	52
over 1/2 English muffin	1 cup sauce	313	130	42
Chicken and dumplings, with 1 dumpling	3 oz meat	255	81	32
frozen (Banquet)	7 oz	280	126	45
Chicken and rice soup	1 cup	48	11	23
Chicken basket (Skipper's)				
5 strips and fries	1 basket	793	342	43
3 strips, 1 fish fillet and fries	1 basket	804	360	45
3 strips, original shrimp and fries	1 basket	800	351	44
Chicken Burrito, frozen (Weight Watchers)	7.62 oz	330	126	38
Chicken Cacciatore				
1/2 breast	1 serving	235	126	54
with 1/2 cup rice ✔	4 oz meat	327	99	30
frozen (Budget Gourmet)	11 oz	300	117	39
Chicken Chow Mein, frozen (Stouffer's)	8 oz	140	45	32
Chicken consomme or broth	1 cup	22	5	23
condensed	1 cup	44	2	5
Chicken divan ✔	1 cup	337	189	56
Chicken enchiladas ✔	2 each	535	279	52
Chicken franks, 10 = 1 lb	1.6 oz	117	79	68
Chicken fricassee ✔	4 oz meat	376	135	36
frozen (Armour)	11 3/4 oz	340	99	29
Chicken fried round steak ✔	4 oz	363	225	62
Chicken fried steak (Wendy's)	6 oz	580	369	64
Chicken gizzards, simmered	1 gizzard	34	7	21
Chicken, ground, cooked	1 oz	49	30	61
Chicken gumbo soup (Campbell's)	1 cup	52	9	17
Chicken heart, simmered	1 heart	6	2	33

FOOD

CALORIES

	AMOUNT	TOTAL	FAT	%FAT
Chicken in a Biscuit (Nabisco)	1 cracker	10	5	50
Chicken Kiev ✔	4 oz meat	334	171	51
frozen entree (Le Menu)	8 oz	530	351	66
Chicken liver, simmered	1 oz	44	14	32
Chicken livers, with tomato sauce				
and noodles	3 oz meat	351	108	31
Chicken luncheon meat (Land O'Frost)	1 oz	60	36	60
Chicken McNugget sauce (McDonald's)				
barbecue	1 oz	50	5	10
honey	1/2 oz	45	0	0
hot mustard	1 oz	70	32	46
sweet and sour	1 oz	60	2	3
Chicken McNuggets, 4 oz (McDonald's)	1 serving	290	147	50
Chicken 'n pasta salad (Hardee's)	1 salad	230	27	12
Chicken Noodle O's (Campbell's)	1 cup	70	18	26
Chicken noodle soup				
(Campbell's)	1 cup	61	18	30
dry, reconstituted	1 cup	53	11	21
(Progesso)	1 cup	110	29	26
Chicken nugget sauce (Kentucky Fried Chicken)				
barbecue	1 oz	35	5	14
honey	1/2 oz	49	tr	tr
mustard	1 oz	36	8	22
sweet and sour	1 oz	58	5	9
Chicken nuggets (Kentucky Fried Chicken)	1 piece	46	26	56
Chicken nuggets (Wendy's)	6 pieces	310	189	61
Chicken Nuggets, breaded, frozen				
3 oz = 5 nuggets (Swanson)	3 oz	250	144	58
Chicken Nuggets, frozen				
(Banquet Kid Cuisine)	6.25 oz	400	171	43
Chicken Oriental dinner				
frozen (Healthy Choice)	11 1/4 oz	220	18	8
Chicken parmesan ✔	4 oz meat	290	144	50
Chicken Patty, breaded (Country Pride)	3 oz	232	135	58
Chicken Picatta, frozen (Tyson)	9 oz	240	90	38

FOOD

CALORIES

	AMOUNT	TOTAL	FAT	%FAT
Chicken potpie, 5" diameter ✔	1 pie	619	315	51
frozen (Swanson)	7 oz	380	198	52
Chicken salad ✔	1/2 cup	158	72	46
(Burger King)	1 salad	140	36	26
Chicken sandwich	1 sandwich	580	270	47
(Arby's)	1 sandwich	493	225	46
(Dairy Queen)	1 sandwich	670	369	55
Grilled (Hardee's)	1 sandwich	310	81	26
(Hardee's)	1 sandwich	370	117	32
hot, with 3 Tbsp gravy	1 sandwich	356	138	39
Littles (Kentucky Fried Chicken)	1 sandwich	169	90	53
(McDonald's)	1 sandwich	490	257	53
(Skipper's)	1 sandwich	606	288	48
Specialty (Burger King)	1 sandwich	688	360	52
(Wendy's)	1 sandwich	430	171	40
with lettuce on white	1 sandwich	303	126	42
Chicken soup, hearty (Progresso)	1 cup	118	29	25
Chicken stew (Chef Boyardee)	1 cup	160	54	34
Chicken strips (Skipper's)	1 strip	82	36	44
Chicken Tamale Platter, frozen (Swanson)	9 3/4 oz	360	135	38
Chicken tenders (Burger King)	1 serving	204	90	44
Chicken teriyaki ✔	1/2 cup	266	160	60
Chicken teriyaki kebabs ✔	1 kebab	194	36	19
Chicken vegetable-noodle soup ✔	1 cup	295	90	31
Chicken, Chinese				
with almonds	1 cup	408	220	54
with broccoli	1 cup	361	225	62
with cashew nuts	1 cup	408	220	54
with mushrooms	1 cup	328	183	56
Chicken, curried with 3/4 cup vegetables	4 oz meat	462	171	37
Chicken, dark meat				
baked, without skin	1 oz	58	25	43
cubes, baked, without skin	1/2 cup	123	39	32
diced, 1 cup = 4.5 oz	1 cup	261	113	43
fried, without skin, without breading	1 oz	75	35	47
raw, without skin	1 oz	37	12	32

FOOD | CALORIES

	AMOUNT	TOTAL	FAT	%FAT
Chicken, light meat				
baked, without skin	1 oz	47	10	21
cubes, baked, without skin	1/2 cup	116	21	18
diced, 1 cup = 4.5 oz	1 cup	211	45	21
fried, with skin, without breading	1 oz	67	25	37
raw, without skin	1 oz	33	5	15
Chicken, breast, baked				
with skin, 3.5 oz	1 breast	193	68	35
without skin, 3 oz	1 breast	142	30	21
Chicken, drumstick, baked				
with skin, 1.75 oz	1 piece	112	52	46
without skin, 1.5 oz	1 piece	87	37	43
Chicken, thigh, baked				
with skin, 2 oz	1 thigh	153	86	56
without skin, 1.75 oz	1 thigh	109	51	47
Chicken, wing, baked				
with skin, 1 oz	1 wing	99	59	60
without skin, 1/2 oz	1 wing	29	12	41
Chicken, extra crispy, (Kentucky Fried Chicken)				
breast	1 piece	354	213	60
drumstick	1 piece	173	98	57
thigh	1 piece	371	234	63
wing	1 piece	218	140	64
Chicken, original recipe, (Kentucky Fried Chicken)				
breast	1 piece	283	135	48
drumstick	1 piece	146	77	52
thigh	1 piece	294	177	60
wing	1 piece	178	105	59
Chicken, boned, canned	1 oz	57	30	53
Chicken, Breast of, Marsala				
frozen (Lean Cuisine)	8 1/8 oz	190	45	24
Chicken, breast, batter fried	1 breast	364	167	46
Chicken, fried ✔	4 oz meat	218	99	45
Chicken, stewed	4 oz meat	167	54	32

FOOD

CALORIES

	AMOUNT	TOTAL	FAT	%FAT
Chicken-stuffed tomato ✔	1 salad	338	225	67
Chickpeas, garbanzo or ceci beans				
cooked	1 cup	338	41	12
dry	1 cup	720	86	12
Chiffon cake, 1/12 of 10" tube ✔	1 piece	287	109	38
Chili (Wendy's)	1 cup	230	81	35
Chili con carne				
homemade ✔	1 cup	481	225	47
with beans, canned (Stokley)	1 cup	390	234	60
without beans, canned (Stokely)	1 cup	430	315	73
Chili dog (Dairy Queen)	1 serving	320	180	56
Chili powder	1 tsp	5	tr	tr
Chili relleno, with cheese, fried ✔	1 serving	146	95	65
Chili, chicken, with beans, Lite (Dennison's)	1 cup	224	45	20
Chili, meatless ✔	1 cup	260	28	11
Chili, with beans, Lite (Dennison's)	1 cup	213	45	21
Chilies, green	1 Tbsp	4	0	0
Chinese beef with tomato ✔	1 cup	265	198	75
Chinese cabbage				
cooked	1/2 cup	12	tr	tr
raw	1/2 cup	6	tr	tr
Chinese chicken				
with almonds	1 cup	408	220	54
with broccoli	1 cup	361	225	62
with cashew nuts	1 cup	408	220	54
with mushrooms	1 cup	328	183	56
Chinese fortune cookies	1 cookie	66	36	55
Chipped beef ✔				
creamed	1 cup	357	228	64
with 3.8% milk	1 cup	274	135	49
with skim milk	1 cup	243	104	43
Chocolate bar, large size, 8 oz (Hershey)	1 bar	1200	648	54
regular size, 1.5 oz (Hershey)	1 bar	220	117	53
with almonds	1 bar	230	126	55

FOOD | CALORIES

	AMOUNT	TOTAL	FAT	%FAT
Chocolate chip cookie				
3" diameter	1 cookie	65	32	49
Almost Home (Nabisco)	1 cookie	60	27	45
Big Batch mix	1 cookie	120	54	45
36 cookies	1 pkg	4320	1944	45
commercial, 1 3/4" diameter	1 small	34	14	41
(Dunkin' Donuts)	1 cookie	129	63	49
(McDonald's)	1 box	330	140	43
(Wendy's)	1 cookie	320	153	48
Chocolate chips, 1 pkg	12 oz	1720	1024	60
3 oz = 1/2 cup	1/2 cup	430	256	60
Chocolate fudge cake				
without frosting (Betty Crocker)	1 cake	3000	1188	40
1/12, with 3 Tbsp frosting	1 piece	436	165	38
1/12, without frosting (Betty Crocker)	1 piece	250	99	40
Chocolate, Lights, snack size (Hostess)	1.25 oz	110	9	8
Chocolate coated creams, 1 piece = 1/2 oz	1 piece	57	20	35
Chocolate coated nougat with carmel	1 oz	118	35	30
Chocolate coated peanuts	1 oz	160	101	63
Chocolate covered cherries	1 oz	126	36	29
Chocolate covered coconut, candy	1 oz	124	45	36
Chocolate cream pie ✔				
1/6 of 9"	1 piece	360	156	43
1/8 of 9"	1 piece	270	117	43
9", whole	1 pie	2160	936	43
Chocolate meringue pie ✔				
1/6 of 9"	1 piece	382	164	43
1/8 of 9"	1 piece	287	123	43
9", whole	1 pie	2293	983	43
Chocolate milk				
1%	1 cup	160	26	16
2%, lowfat	1 cup	180	45	25
3.8%, whole	1 cup	210	72	34
Chocolate Mint Treat (Weight Watchers)				
1 = 2.7 oz	1 serving	100	9	9

FOOD | CALORIES

	AMOUNT	TOTAL	FAT	%FAT
Chocolate syrup				
(Hershey)	1 Tbsp	53	2	4
fudge type	1 Tbsp	62	23	37
thin type	1 Tbsp	46	4	9
Chocolate, bitter or baking	1 oz	142	135	95
Chop suey, with meat canned	1 cup	223	103	46
Chorizo, pork and beef	2 oz link	265	207	78
Chow mein noodles, hard, canned	1 cup	220	108	49
Chow mein				
Chicken, frozen (Stouffer's)	8 oz	140	45	32
chicken, without noodles	1 cup	255	90	35
shrimp, without noodles	1 cup	221	90	41
vegetable, frozen (La Choy)	1 cup	69	3	4
Chunky chicken salad (McDonald's)	1 salad	140	31	22
Cider, apple	8 oz	123	0	0
Cilantro	10 sprigs	2	tr	tr
Cider, apple	8 oz	123	0	0
Cinnamon Crispas (Taco Bell)	1 serving	259	138	53
Cinnamon roll, plain, small				
3" diameter (Pillsbury)	1 roll	145	56	39
homemade ✔	1 roll	176	45	26
Clam chowder				
Manhattan (Campbell's)	1 cup	70	9	13
New England				
3.8% milk (Campbell's)	1 cup	157	54	34
with water (Campbell's)	1 cup	77	18	23
(Skipper's)	1 cup	100	32	32
Clam juice	1 cup	6	tr	tr
Clams				
breaded, fried ✔	1 oz	57	28	49
steamed or canned	1 oz	42	5	12
Club sandwich, chicken (Arby's)	1 sandwich	610	297	49
Club Soda (Schweppes)	12 oz	tr	0	0
Cobbler, apple ✔	3/4 cup	505	198	39
Coca Cola	12 oz	144	0	0
Cocktail sauce ✔	1 Tbsp	15	0	0

FOOD

CALORIES

	AMOUNT	TOTAL	FAT	%FAT
Cocoa, baking	1 Tbsp	21	15	71
Cocoa, instant				
reconstituted with water (Swiss Miss)	8 oz	146	36	25
sugar free, reconstituted (Swiss Miss)	8 oz	64	0	0
sugar free, reconstituted (Alba)	8 oz	60	0	0
with marshmallow, reconstituted				
with water	8 oz	146	36	25
with powdered skim milk	4 tsp	109	9	8
Coconut cream pie ✔				
1/6 of 9"	1 piece	697	324	46
1/8 of 9"	1 piece	523	243	46
9", whole	1 pie	4184	1944	46
Coconut				
dried, shredded, 2.2 oz	1 cup	344	218	63
fresh, 1 x 1 x 3/8"	1 piece	54	47	87
shredded, 3.4 oz	1 cup	349	303	87
Cod				
broiled or baked	1 oz	30	2	7
(Skipper's)	1 piece	94	41	44
3 pieces with fries	1 basket	665	288	43
Coffee roll, honey dipped (Dunkin' Donuts)	1 roll	348	153	44
Coffee, instant granules	1 tsp	4	0	0
Coffee, regular or decaffeinated	6 oz	4	tr	tr
Coffeecake, 2 3/4" square	1 piece	230	62	27
8 x 5 1/2 x 1 1/4"	1 cake	1385	361	26
Cola type beverages	12 oz	145	0	0
Colby cheese	1 oz	112	82	73
Coleslaw				
with mayonnaise-type dressing	1/2 cup	103	88	85
(Kentucky Fried Chicken)	1 serving	119	59	50
(Skipper's)	1/2 cup	289	243	84
Coleslaw dressing	1 Tbsp	70	54	77
Collards, fresh or frozen, cooked	1/2 cup	33	4	12
Coney Island ✔	1 sandwich	373	225	60
Consomme	1 cup	29	0	0
Cookie dough, plain, chilled roll, 18 oz	1 roll	2290	1037	45

FOOD		CALORIES		
	AMOUNT	TOTAL	FAT	%FAT
Cookies 'n Cream sandwich (Oreo)	1 bar	240	99	41
Cool Whip topping	1 Tbsp	12	9	75
	1 cup	192	144	75
Extra Creamy	1 Tbsp	16	11	69
	1 cup	256	176	69
Lite	1 Tbsp	8	6	75
	1 cup	128	96	75
Corn Chex (Ralston)	1 cup	110	0	0
Corn candy	1/2 cup	364	18	5
Corn chips				
10 chips = 1 oz (Tostitos)	1 oz	150	72	48
15 chips = 1 oz (Doritos)	1 oz	140	56	40
15 chips = 1 oz (Frito Lay)	1 oz	160	90	56
Corn dog	1 serving	345	202	59
Corn Flakes (Kellogg's)	1 cup	100	0	0
Corn fritters ✔	1 oz	62	18	29
Corn muffin, 3" diameter	1 muffin	215	92	43
4" diameter	1 muffin	287	122	43
(Dunkin' Donuts)	1 muffin	347	117	34
Corn nuts, snack food	1 oz	110	27	25
Corn on the cob				
fresh or frozen, 5" ear	1 ear	118	11	9
(Kentucky Fried Chicken)	1 piece	176	28	16
Corn syrup, light and dark, (Karo)	1 Tbsp	55	0	0
Corn, sweet				
canned or frozen, cooked	1/2 cup	70	4	6
canned, cream style	1/2 cup	105	9	9
in butter sauce, frozen	3.3 oz	90	18	20
Cornbread, 3" square ✔	1 piece	193	60	31
from mix, 1/12 pkg (General Mills)	1 piece	160	45	28
Corned beef hash	1 cup	398	224	56
Corned beef sandwich on rye	1 sandwich	377	182	48
Corned beef, boneless				
canned	1 oz	61	31	51
cooked	1 oz	71	48	68

FOOD

CALORIES

	AMOUNT	TOTAL	FAT	%FAT
Cornish game hen				
baked, without skin	1 oz	40	10	25
raw, with skin	1 whole	400	198	50
Cornmeal, yellow or white				
cooked	1 cup	120	5	4
dry	1 cup	530	16	3
Cornstarch	1 Tbsp	29	0	0
Cottage cheese				
1% fat, all curds	1/2 cup	83	9	11
2% fat, all curds	1/2 cup	103	18	17
4% fat, all curds	1/2 cup	118	44	37
dry curd	1/2 cup	63	5	8
Couscous, cooked	1 cup	160	0	0
Cowpeas or blackeyed peas				
cooked	1 cup	178	12	7
raw	1 cup	184	10	5
Crab apples, fresh, sliced	1/2 cup	68	3	4
Crab cocktail	2 oz	52	9	17
Crab Louis ✔	1 salad	642	495	77
Crab meat, imitation	1 oz	29	3	10
Crab stuffed chicken breasts ✔	1/2 breast	449	135	30
Crab				
Alaska King, steamed	1 oz	27	4	15
Blue, canned	1 oz	28	3	11
Dungeness				
steamed	1 oz	26	5	19
flaked	1 cup	116	21	18
pieces	1 cup	144	26	18
White, canned	1 oz	29	6	21
	1 cup	135	26	19
Cracked wheat bread, 4 1/2 x 4 1/2"	1 slice	65	8	12
Cracked wheat crackers				
(Pepperidge Farm)	1 cracker	28	9	32
Cracklebred (Jacquet)	1 cracker	17	tr	tr
Cracklin' Oat Bran (Kellogg's)	1 cup	220	72	33

FOOD		CALORIES		
	AMOUNT	TOTAL	FAT	%FAT
Cran-raspberry juice,				
bottled (Ocean Spray)	8 oz	144	tr	tr
Cranapple juice, bottled (Ocean Spray)	8 oz	168	tr	tr
Cranberries, fresh, whole	1/2 cup	22	3	14
Cranberry apple juice, bottled	8 oz	172	2	1
Cranberry juice				
bottled, sweetened	8 oz	165	1	1
low calorie, bottled	8 oz	48	4	8
Cranberry orange relish ✔	1 Tbsp	27	1	4
Cranberry sauce, canned, sweetened	1/4 cup	102	2	2
Cream cheese				
Light, Philadelphia	1 oz	60	45	75
Philadelphia	1 oz	100	90	90
Philadelphia, soft tub	2 Tbsp	100	90	90
reduced fat, Neufchatel	1 oz	74	58	78
Cream of broccoli soup ✔	1 cup	169	99	59
Cream of celery soup (Campbell's)				
with 3.8% milk	1 cup	181	94	52
with skim milk	1 cup	143	54	38
with water	1 cup	86	44	51
Cream of chicken soup				
homemade ✔	1 cup	282	162	57
condensed	1 cup	218	126	58
with 3.8% milk	1 cup	189	94	50
with skim milk	1 cup	152	54	36
with water	1 cup	109	54	50
dry, reconstituted	1 cup	107	48	45
Cream of mushroom soup				
condensed	1 cup	194	108	56
with 3.8% milk	1 cup	178	94	53
with skim milk	1 cup	140	54	39
with water	1 cup	97	54	56
Cream of potato soup				
homemade ✔	1 cup	191	91	48
with water (Campbell's)	1 cup	70	27	39
Cream of Rice, cooked	1 cup	160	tr	tr

FOOD		CALORIES		
	AMOUNT	TOTAL	FAT	%FAT
Cream of tomato soup ✔	1 cup	189	99	52
Cream of Wheat, cooked	1 cup	133	4	3
Cream puff				
shell, 3 1/2 x 2" ✔	1 shell	156	105	67
with custard filling	1 average	303	163	54
with whipped cream filling ✔	1 average	279	216	77
Cream				
half-and-half	1 Tbsp	20	17	85
	1 cup	320	272	85
light	1 Tbsp	30	28	93
	1 cup	480	448	93
whipping, heavy, unwhipped	1 Tbsp	53	50	94
	1 cup	848	800	94
whipped	1 Tbsp	26	25	96
	1 cup	416	400	96
Creamer, dry				
Coffee Mate (Carnation)	1 Tbsp	30	27	90
Lite	1 Tbsp	24	18	75
Cremora (Borden)	1 Tbsp	36	27	75
Creamer, imitation, liquid				
(Carnation)	1 Tbsp	33	18	55
(Mocha Mix)	1 Tbsp	20	18	90
Creamsicle (Sealtest)	1 average	103	28	27
Creamy cucumber dressing	1 Tbsp	70	63	90
reduced calorie	1 Tbsp	25	18	72
Creme DeMenthe	1 oz	101	0	0
Crepe				
without filling, 6" diameter	1 crepe	58	24	41
Suzette ✔	2 crepes	334	144	43
with shrimp filling (Mrs. Smith's)	2 crepes	305	144	47
with strawberry filling (Mrs. Smith's)	1 crepe	150	45	30
Crispbread, High Fiber (Ryvita)	1 cracker	23	tr	tr
Crispix (Kellogg's)	1 cup	110	0	0
Crispy Curls (Hardee's)	1 serving	300	144	48
Crispy Wheat and Raisins (General Mills)	1 cup	145	12	8

FOOD

CALORIES

	AMOUNT	TOTAL	FAT	%FAT
Croissant				
frozen, 1 oz (Sara Lee)	1 small	109	55	50
1.5 oz (Sara Lee)	1 medium	170	81	48
homemade ✔	1 small	100	54	54
plain (Dunkin' Donuts)	1 croissant	291	198	68
almond	1 croissant	435	270	62
chocolate	1 croissant	502	333	66
Croissanwich, breakfast (Burger King)				
bacon	1 sandwich	355	216	61
ham	1 sandwich	335	180	54
sausage	1 sandwich	538	369	69
Croutons	1 Tbsp	37	2	5
Cruller, French, with glaze (Dunkin' Donuts)	1 donut	201	126	63
honey dipped	1 donut	370	207	56
Crumpet, 3" diameter	1 roll	129	27	21
Cucumber, raw	1 medium	16	2	13
Cupcake, plain, from mix,				
2 1/2" diameter	1 cupcake	88	27	31
Curacao, orange flavored liqueur	1 oz	81	0	0
Currants, dried	1/4 cup	100	4	4
Curried chicken salad ✔	1 cup	582	288	49
Curried rice ✔	1/2 cup	233	54	23
Curry sauce ✔	1 Tbsp	26	18	69
Custard pie ✔				
1/6 of 9"	1 piece	401	196	49
1/8 of 9"	1 piece	301	147	49
9", whole	1 pie	2408	1174	49
Custard, baked with 3.8% milk ✔	1/2 cup	153	66	43
Custard pudding				
with 2% milk (Jell-O)	1/2 cup	153	30	20
with skim milk (Jell-O)	1/2 cup	133	9	7

FOOD

CALORIES

	AMOUNT	TOTAL	FAT	%FAT

D

	AMOUNT	TOTAL	FAT	%FAT
Daiquiri	3 oz	122	0	0
Dandelion greens	1/2 cup	18	4	22
Danish				
apple, frozen (Sara Lee)	1 roll	360	122	34
caramel, refrigerated (Pillsbury)	1 roll	157	68	43
cheese, frozen (Sara Lee)	1 roll	308	151	49
great (Burger King)	1 roll	500	324	65
(McDonald's)				
apple	1 roll	390	161	41
cinnamon raisin	1 roll	440	189	43
iced cheese	1 roll	390	196	50
raspberry	1 roll	410	143	35
(Wendy's)				
apple	1 roll	360	126	35
cheese	1 roll	430	189	44
cinnamon raisin	1 roll	410	162	40
Dates				
chopped	1/2 cup	245	4	2
whole, without pits	1 date	22	tr	tr
Devil's Food cake				
1/12, with 3 Tbsp 7 minute frosting	1 piece	395	108	27
1/12, with frosting (Betty Crocker)	1 piece	260	108	42
cupcake, 2 1/2" diameter, plain	1 cupcake	120	34	28
without frosting (Betty Crocker)	1 cake	3120	1296	42
Deviled ham, canned	1 Tbsp	45	36	80
Dill sauce ✔	1/4 cup	18	9	50
Dilly bar (Dairy Queen)	1 serving	210	117	56
Dim Sum, 4 oz ✔	1 roll	345	189	55
Ding dong, 1 1/2" diameter (Hostess)	1 piece	187	95	51
Dinner rolls ✔	1 roll	98	27	28

FOOD	AMOUNT	CALORIES		
		TOTAL	FAT	%FAT
Donut, cake, iced or sugared, 3 1/4" diameter	1 average	184	71	39
Donut, cake (Dunkin' Donuts)				
chocolate with glaze	1 donut	324	189	58
coconut coated	1 donut	417	252	60
Munchkin with powdered sugar	1 donut	69	36	52
Munchkin chocolate with glaze	1 donut	88	45	51
plain	1 donut	319	198	62
Donut, filled (Dunkin' Donuts)				
apple with cinnamon sugar	1 donut	219	108	49
Bavarian creme	1 donut	226	126	56
with chocolate frosting	1 donut	231	81	35
blueberry	1 donut	196	90	46
jelly	1 donut	274	198	72
lemon	1 donut	221	99	45
Donut, plain				
1 1/2" diameter	1 donut	55	23	42
2 1/2" diameter	1 donut	98	41	42
3 1/4" diameter	1 donut	164	69	42
3 5/8" diameter	1 donut	227	95	42
Donut, raised or yeast				
cream filled, 3 1/2" diameter	1 average	244	85	35
plain, 3 1/4" diameter	1 average	174	100	57
jelly, 3 1/2" diameter	1 average	226	79	35
Donut, yeast (Dunkin' Donuts)				
chocolate frosted	1 donut	246	126	51
honey dipped	1 donut	208	99	48
Munchkin with glaze	1 donut	43	18	42
sugar jelly stick	1 donut	332	162	49
Doo Dads snack mix	1/2 cup	140	54	39
Dove Bar, 3.8 oz	1 bar	306	135	44
Light	1 bar	230	99	43
DQ sandwich	1 sandwich	140	36	26
Drumstick, ice cream cone	1 average	186	89	48

FOOD		CALORIES		
	AMOUNT	TOTAL	FAT	%FAT
Duck, domestic				
raw, without skin	1 oz	38	15	39
roasted, with skin	1 oz	95	72	76
without skin	1 oz	57	29	51
Dumpling, 2" diameter ✔	1 dumpling	48	29	60

E

	AMOUNT	TOTAL	FAT	%FAT
Eclair with chocolate icing				
custard filling	1 average	263	135	51
pudding filling ✔	1 average	290	135	47
Edam cheese	1 oz	101	70	69
Egg and sausage casserole ✔	1 cup	663	495	75
Egg bread ✔	1 slice	119	18	15
Egg flower soup, Chinese	1 cup	59	27	46
Egg foo yung	1 cup	257	160	62
Egg McMuffin (McDonald's)	1 serving	290	101	35
Egg roll				
chicken, frozen (La Choy)	3 rolls	69	26	38
frozen, restaurant style	3 oz	180	54	30
shrimp, frozen (La Choy)	3 rolls	62	21	34
Egg salad ✔	1/2 cup	307	249	81
Egg substitute				
(Second Nature)	1/4 cup	53	24	45
frozen (Egg Beaters)	1/4 cup	25	0	0
(Morning Star Farms)	1/4 cup	60	27	45

FOOD

CALORIES

	AMOUNT	TOTAL	FAT	%FAT
Egg				
hard/soft boiled, without fat	1 egg	75	45	60
omelet, plain, 2 eggs	1 serving	189	128	68
poached, without fat	1 egg	75	45	60
poached/fried with 1 tsp fat	1 egg	109	79	72
Egg, raw, large				
white	1 white	17	tr	tr
whole	1 egg	75	45	60
yolk	1 yolk	58	45	78
Egg, turkey, raw, whole	1 medium	135	85	63
Eggnog				
(4 oz) with 1 oz rum	5 oz	245	85	35
(nonalcoholic)	8 oz	340	171	50
Eggplant				
cooked	1/2 cup	19	2	11
parmigiana ✔	1 cup	336	155	46
Eggs Benedict ✔	1 serving	465	324	70
Eggs				
deviled ✔	2 halves	145	116	80
scrambled (McDonald's)	1 serving	140	88	63
Elderberries, fresh	1/2 cup	72	5	7
Enchilada dinner, frozen (Swanson)				
beef	13 3/4 oz	480	198	41
chicken	9 oz	290	90	31
Enchilada sauce, mild or hot (Del Monte)	1/2 cup	39	1	3
Enchilada				
beef ✔	6 oz	317	187	59
cheese ✔	6 oz	320	170	53
chicken ✔	6 0z	240	68	28
Enchiladas, frozen (El Charrito)				
beef	11 oz	560	279	50
cheese	11 oz	470	180	38
chicken	11 oz	440	117	27
Enchirito (Taco Bell)	1 serving	382	177	46
Endive, small pieces	1 cup	10	tr	tr

FOOD

CALORIES

	AMOUNT	TOTAL	FAT	%FAT
English muffin	1 muffin	160	9	6
cinnamon raisin	1 muffin	170	9	5
oat nut bran	1 muffin	160	18	11
sourdough	1 muffin	140	9	6
buttered (McDonald's)	1 muffin	170	41	24
English Water Biscuit (Pepperidge Farm)	1 cracker	18	2	11
Eskimo Pie, 3 oz	1 bar	180	108	60
Light, 2.5 oz	1 bar	140	80	57
Sugar free, 2.5 oz	1 bar	140	108	77
Evaporated milk				
skim	8 oz	200	9	5
whole	8 oz	340	171	50

F

	AMOUNT	TOTAL	FAT	%FAT
Fajita (Taco Bell)				
chicken	1 serving	226	92	41
steak	1 serving	233	98	42
Farina, quick cook or regular, cooked	1 cup	105	2	2
Farmer's cheese	1 oz	90	63	70
Fava or broad beans, dry	1 lb	1533	69	5
Feta cheese	1 oz	75	53	71
Fettuccini Alfredo ✔	1 cup	550	306	57
Fettuccini, noodles				
cooked	1 cup	150	9	6
dry	1 cup	200	9	5

FOOD

CALORIES

	AMOUNT	TOTAL	FAT	%FAT
Fettuccini, spinach				
cooked	1 cup	150	9	6
dry	1 cup	200	9	5
Fig bar cookie, 1 5/8 x 3/8" square	1 cookie	50	6	12
Figs, canned, whole				
in heavy syrup	1/2 cup	109	3	3
water pack	1/2 cup	60	2	3
Figs, fresh				
1 1/2" diameter	1 fig	32	1	3
2 1/4" diameter	1 fig	40	2	5
Filberts or Hazelnuts, whole				
20 = 1 oz	1 oz	183	161	88
4.8 oz = 1 cup	1 cup	878	773	88
Filet-0-Fish sandwich (McDonald's)	1 sandwich	440	235	53
Fish 'n Chips dinner, frozen (Swanson)	10 oz	500	180	36
Fish 'n Chips, frozen				
1 fillet = 3 1/4 oz (Swanson)	3 1/4 oz	175	77	44
Fish Creole ✔	4 oz fish	351	108	31
Fish fillet, breaded, fried (Skipper's)	2.5 oz	175	90	51
Fish Fillets, battered, frozen				
1 fillet = 2 1/2 oz (Van de Kamp's)	2 1/2 oz	170	81	48
Fish Florentine ✔	4 oz fish	240	108	45
Fish sandwich				
(Dairy Queen)	1 sandwich	400	153	38
with cheese (Dairy Queen)	1 sandwich	440	189	43
(Hardee's)	1 sandwich	500	216	43
(Skipper's)	1 sandwich	524	297	57
double (Skipper's)	1 sandwich	698	657	94
(Wendy's)	1 sandwich	210	99	47
Fish Sticks, breaded, frozen (Van de Kamp's)	4 sticks	190	90	47
Flan	1/2 cup	180	79	44
Float (Dairy Queen)	1 serving	410	63	15
Flounder				
broiled	1 oz	33	4	12
stuffed ✔	4 oz fish	311	153	49

FOOD		CALORIES		
	AMOUNT	TOTAL	FAT	%FAT
Flour				
all-purpose, white	1 Tbsp	29	1	3
	1 cup	400	10	3
barley	1 Tbsp	28	1	4
	1 cup	401	17	4
buckwheat, light or dark	1 Tbsp	22	1	5
	1 cup	347	11	3
gluten	1 Tbsp	33	2	6
	1 cup	529	24	5
potato	1 Tbsp	22	tr	tr
	1 cup	351	7	2
rice	1 Tbsp	30	tr	tr
	1 cup	479	4	1
rye, dark	1 Tbsp	27	2	7
	1 cup	419	26	6
rye, light	1 Tbsp	20	1	5
	1 cup	314	8	3
soybean, low-fat	1 Tbsp	19	3	16
	1 cup	304	48	16
whole wheat	1 Tbsp	29	1	3
	1 cup	400	22	6
Fontina cheese	1 oz	110	77	70
Fortune cookie, Chinese	1 cookie	66	36	55
Freeze (Dairy Queen)	1 serving	500	108	22
French bread, 5 x 2 1/2 x 1"	1 slice	100	8	8
French dip sandwich, 3 oz meat	1 sandwich	461	248	54
French fries				
frozen, oven heated	10 pieces	110	34	31
2.5 oz (Arby's)	1 serving	246	119	48
regular (Burger King)	1 serving	227	117	52
large (Dairy Queen)	1 serving	320	144	45
regular (Dairy Queen)	1 serving	200	90	45
regular (Hardee's)	1 serving	230	99	43
(Kentucky Fried Chicken)	1 serving	244	107	44
large (McDonald"s)	1 serving	400	194	49

FOOD

CALORIES

	AMOUNT	TOTAL	FAT	%FAT
French Fries (continued)				
regular (McDonald's)	1 serving	320	154	48
small (McDonald's)	1 serving	220	108	49
(Skipper's)	1 sering	383	162	42
3 oz (Wendy's)	1 serving	300	135	45
French onion soup ✔	1 cup	283	108	38
French salad dressing	1 Tbsp	65	53	82
reduced calorie	1 Tbsp	15	9	60
(Burger King)	1 packet	280	207	74
(McDonald's)	1 packet	230	187	81
red (McDonald's)	1 packet	160	68	43
French toast				
4 1/2 x 4 1/2" ✔	1 slice	119	30	25
4 x 4" (Aunt Jemima)	1 slice	56	15	27
frozen (Eggo)	1 slice	72	17	24
(Wendy's)	2 slices	400	171	43
with apple topping	2 slices	530	171	32
with blueberry topping	2 slices	460	171	37
French toast sticks (Burger King)	1 serving	499	261	52
Fresh fruit cup	1 cup	104	tr	tr
Fried Chicken dinner, frozen (Banquet)	10 oz	400	180	45
Fried Chicken, Original, frozen (Banquet)	6.4 oz	330	171	52
Hot 'n Spicy	6.4 oz	330	171	52
Fried Rice, frozen (Chun King)				
with chicken	8 oz	260	36	14
with pork	8 oz	270	54	20
Fried rice, with pork				
(Chun King)	1 cup	144	57	40
Chinese ✔	1 cup	312	166	53
Frosted Mini Wheats (Kellogg's)	1 cup	200	0	0
Frosting				
butter with powdered sugar ✔	1 Tbsp	60	17	28
	1 cup	944	272	29
chocolate and vanilla, Ready to Spread	1 Tbsp	60	24	40
	16 oz	1920	756	39
chocolate fudge ✔	1 Tbsp	62	22	35

FOOD		CALORIES		
	AMOUNT	TOTAL	FAT	%FAT
Frosting (continued)				
cream cheese with nuts,				
mix (Betty Crocker)	1 Tbsp	75	27	36
	1 pkg	1800	648	36
cream cheese				
homemade ✔	1 Tbsp	63	20	32
Ready to Spread	1 Tbsp	64	24	38
	16 oz	2040	756	37
German chocolate ✔	1 Tbsp	70	50	71
seven minute ✔	1 Tbsp	45	0	0
Frosty dairy dessert (Wendy's)				
large	20 oz	666	210	32
medium	16 oz	533	168	32
small	12 oz	400	126	32
Frozen dessert, all flavor,				
7 x 3 1/2 x 1/2" (Weight Watchers)	1 slice	100	36	36
Frozen bread dough				
honey wheat (Rhodes)	1/14 loaf	75	5	7
	1 loaf	1050	63	6
white (Rhodes)	1/14 loaf	80	5	7
	1 loaf	1120	63	6
Frozen dinner roll, white (Rhodes)	1 roll	85	27	32
Fruit and Cream Bar (Chiquita)	1 bar	80	9	11
Fruit and Juice Bar, 2.5 oz (Dole)	1 bar	70	tr	tr
Fresh Lites, 1.65 oz	1 bar	25	tr	tr
Fruit and Yogurt Bar (Dole)	1 bar	70	tr	tr
Fruit and Fiber, all varieties (Post)	1 cup	180	18	10
Fruit Loops (Kellogg's)	1 cup	110	9	8
Fruit Muesli (Ralston)	1 cup	300	54	18
Fruit cocktail, canned				
in heavy syrup	1/2 cup	76	1	1
juice pack	1/2 cup	50	1	2
water pack	1/2 cup	37	1	3
Fruit Gems (Sunkist)	1 waffer	31	tr	tr
Fruit Punch (Hawaiian Punch)	8 oz	120	tr	tr
"lite" (Hawaiian Punch)	8 oz	107	tr	tr

FOOD

CALORIES

	AMOUNT	TOTAL	FAT	%FAT
Fruit-flavored carbonated sodas	12 oz	166	0	0
sugar free	12 oz	3	0	0
Fruitcake ✔				
dark, 7" diameter	1 cake	5216	1888	36
dark, 1/16 of 7" diameter	1 piece	326	118	36
light	1/36 cake	234	72	31
Fudge Cakes, snack size (Sara Lee)	1 cake	190	90	47
Fudge, chocolate, with walnuts, 1" cube	1 piece	89	33	37
Fudgsicle, 1.75 oz	1 bar	70	9	13
sugar free, 1.25 oz	1 bar	35	9	26

G

	AMOUNT	TOTAL	FAT	%FAT
Garbanzo, chickpeas, ceci beans				
cooked	1 cup	338	41	12
dry	1 cup	720	86	12
Garden salad				
(Burger King)	1 salad	90	45	50
(Hardee's)	1 salad	210	126	60
(McDonald's)	1 salad	110	59	54
(Wendy's)	1 salad	102	45	44
Gardenburger, vegetable patty	1/4 lb	147	46	31
Garlic bread ✔	2 slices	145	81	56
Garlic clove, raw	1 clove	4	tr	tr
Gazpacho ✔	1 cup	186	108	58
Gefiltefish, sweet	1 oz	18	5	28
Gelatin salad, with fruit, sweetened	1/2 cup	80	1	1

FOOD		CALORIES		
	AMOUNT	TOTAL	FAT	%FAT
Gelatin				
dry	1 Tbsp	34	tr	tr
sugar free, all flavors (Jell-O)	1/2 cup	8	0	0
with sugar, all flavors (Jell-O)	1/2 cup	80	0	0
German chocolate cake				
1/12, without frosting (Betty Crocker)	1 piece	260	99	38
1/12, with 3 Tbsp frosting	1 piece	470	249	53
without frosting (Betty Crocker)	1 cake	3120	1188	38
German Stollen ✔	1 slice	94	27	29
Giblet gravy ✔	1/4 cup	47	9	19
Gin, 86 proof	1 oz	70	0	0
Ginger ale (Schweppes)	12 oz	132	0	0
sugar free (Schweppes)	12 oz	4	0	0
Gingerbread, plain				
1/9 of 8" square	1 piece	175	34	19
8" square	1 cake	1575	306	19
Gingersnap cookie, 3" diameter	1 cookie	34	6	18
Gise, frozen dessert	1 cup	76	tr	tr
Gjetost cheese	1 oz	132	74	56
Gnocchi, cheese, baked ✔	1 cup	449	261	58
Golden cake (Betty Crocker)				
1/12, without frosting	1 piece	200	72	36
whole, without frosting	1 cake	2400	864	36
Golden Grahams (General Mills)	1 cup	146	12	8
Goldfish crackers (Pepperidge Farm)	1 oz	136	51	38
Goose, baked, with skin	1 oz	86	56	65
without skin	1 oz	67	32	48
Gooseberries, fresh	1/2 cup	30	1	3
Gouda cheese	1 oz	101	69	68
Graham cracker crumbs	1 Tbsp	29	6	21
	1 cup	462	98	21
Graham cracker crust, 8"	1 crust	1125	646	57
Graham cracker				
chocolate covered	1 square	60	27	45
plain	1 square	30	5	16
snacks, Teddy Grahams, 11 = 1/2 oz	1/2 oz	60	18	30

FOOD

CALORIES

	AMOUNT	TOTAL	FAT	%FAT
Granola				
100% Natural (Quaker Oats)	1 cup	560	212	38
coconut-cashew	1 cup	560	216	39
honey	1 cup	440	144	33
plain (Nature Valley)	1 cup	390	189	48
with cinnamon, raisins (Nature Valley)	1 cup	512	176	34
Granola bar (Nature Valley)				
chewey	1 bar	140	63	45
plain	1 bar	110	36	33
with fruit	1 bar	150	45	30
Grape drink, canned	8 oz	135	tr	tr
Grape juice				
canned, bottled or frozen				
reconstitued	8 oz	165	tr	tr
frozen, concentrate, sweetened	6 oz	395	tr	tr
Grape Nuts, 1 cup = 4 oz (Post)	1 cup	440	tr	tr
Grapefruit				
canned, sweetened	1/2 cup	70	1	1
canned, unsweetened	1/2 cup	30	1	3
fresh, pink, 3 3/4" diameter	1/2 fruit	50	tr	tr
fresh, white, 3 3/4" diameter	1/2 fruit	45	tr	tr
Grapefruit juice				
canned, sweetened	8 oz	135	tr	tr
fresh or frozen, unsweetened,				
reconstituted	8 oz	100	tr	tr
frozen, concentrate	6 oz	300	8	3
Grapes, fresh, all varieties	10 grapes	40	tr	tr
Grasshopper cocktail with cream	3 oz	264	158	60
Gravy				
beef, canned	1/4 cup	31	13	42
beef, with fat drippings ✔	1/4 cup	164	126	77
brown, dry, mix, reconstituted	1/4 cup	2	1	50
chicken or turkey ✔	1/4 cup	128	97	76
chicken, canned	1/4 cup	47	31	66
sausage (Wendy's)	6 oz	440	324	74
turkey, dry, mix, reconstituted	1/4 cup	22	5	23

FOOD

CALORIES

	AMOUNT	TOTAL	FAT	%FAT
Great Northern beans, white				
cooked	1 cup	212	10	5
dry	1 cup	612	26	4
Greek salad ✔	1 salad	429	342	80
Green beans, cut, fresh cooked,				
canned or frozen	1/2 cup	15	tr	tr
Green chilies (Old El Paso)	1 oz	7	0	0
Green onions, scallions, raw, 3/8" diameter	1 onion	3	tr	tr
Green or red pepper, bell				
chopped	2 Tbsp	3	tr	tr
raw	1 large	22	2	9
Green pea soup, with water (Campbell's)	1 cup	150	9	6
Green River cheese, part skim milk	1 oz	101	66	65
Green salad				
with 1 Tbsp dressing	1 cup	112	73	65
without dressing	1 cup	32	3	9
Grilled cheese sandwich on white	1 sandwich	430	239	56
Grits, cooked	1 cup	125	tr	tr
Grouper, broiled	1 oz	34	3	9
Gruyere cheese	1 oz	117	81	69
Guacamole (Taco Bell)	1 serving	34	21	61
Guacamole dip	1 cup	403	297	74
Guava, fresh, medium	1 guava	62	5	8
Gum drops	1 piece	7	tr	tr
	1 oz	98	3	3

FOOD

CALORIES

	AMOUNT	TOTAL	FAT	%FAT

H

Food	AMOUNT	TOTAL	FAT	%FAT
Haddock, broiled	1 oz	32	2	6
Half-and-half, cream	1 Tbsp	20	17	85
	1 cup	320	272	85
Halibut, broiled	1 oz	40	7	18
smoked	1 oz	33	5	15
Ham and Asparagus Au Gratin				
frozen (Budget Gourmet Slim Selects)	9 oz	280	90	32
Ham and bean vegetable soup	1 cup	126	27	21
Ham and cheese sandwich (Arby's)	1 sandwich	292	123	42
Specialty (Burger King)	1 sandwich	471	207	44
Ham				
cannned				
lean, 4% fat	1 oz	39	12	31
regular, 13% fat	1 oz	64	39	61
luncheon				
extra lean, 5% fat	1 oz	37	9	24
regular, 11% fat	1 oz	52	27	52
picnic, roasted	1 oz	65	32	49
diced, 1 cup = 4.5 oz	1 cup	293	144	49
whole, rosted	1 oz	62	28	45
Ham salad ✔	1/2 cup	287	207	72
Ham salad spread	1 oz	61	40	66
Ham-noodle casserole ✔	1 cup	513	288	56
Hamburger bun, 4" diameter				
plain	1 bun	110	18	16
sesame seed	1 bun	150	18	12
Hamburger				
(Burger King)	1 burger	275	108	39
deluxe (Buger King)	1 burger	322	153	48
double (Dairy Queen)	1 burger	530	252	48
single (Dairy Queen)	1 burger	360	144	40

FOOD

CALORIES

	AMOUNT	TOTAL	FAT	%FAT
Hamburger (continued)				
triple (Dairy Queen)	1 burger	710	405	57
(McDonald's)	1 burger	260	86	33
plain, 1/4 pound (Wendy's)	1 burger	350	144	41
single with everything (Wendy's)	1 burger	430	198	46
small (Wendy's)	1 burger	260	81	31
Hasenpfeffer ✔	4 oz	371	144	39
Hashbrowns,				
(McDonald's)	1 serving	130	66	51
homemade ✔	1/2 cup	177	81	46
frozen, not fried (Ore Ida)	6 oz	130	0	0
Hash Rounds (Hardee's)	1 serving	230	126	55
Havarti	1 oz	117	94	80
Hearty Wheat crackers (Pepperidge Farm)	1 cracker	25	16	64
Herb-garlic sauce ✔	1 Tbsp	27	18	67
Herring, Atrantic				
baked	1 oz	58	30	52
canned in tomato sauce	1 oz	50	27	54
kippered	1 oz	60	33	55
pickled	1 oz	78	54	69
Hi-Ho Deluxe crackers (Sunshine)	1 cracker	20	11	55
Hoagie roll, 11 1/2 x 3"	1 roll	392	37	9
Hollandaise sauce ✔	1 Tbsp	45	42	93
	1/4 cup	180	167	93
Hom Bow				
with chicken, steamed dumpling	1 whole	124	41	33
with pork, steamed dumpling	1 whole	176	70	40
Hominy, cooked	1 cup	146	5	3
raw	1 cup	579	16	3
Honey	1 Tbsp	65	0	0
Honey butter ✔	1 Tbsp	60	48	80
Honey Nut Cherrios (General Mills)	1 cup	147	9	6
Honey Wheat Berry Bread				
3 3/4 x 3 3/4 x 1/2"	1 slice	90	9	10

FOOD | CALORIES

FOOD	AMOUNT	TOTAL	FAT	%FAT
Honeydew, fresh				
6 1/2" diameter, 2" wedge	1 wedge	50	4	8
cubed	1/2 cup	28	2	7
Horseradish sauce, creamy (Kraft)	1 Tbsp	50	45	90
Horseradish, prepared	1 Tbsp	7	tr	tr
Hot buttered rum mix ✔	1/3 cup	360	162	45
Hot caramel sundae (McDonald's)	1 sundae	340	82	24
Hot cross buns	1 average	111	29	26
Hot dog				
5" x 3/4", 10 per lb	1.6 oz	139	109	78
5" x 7/8", 8 per lb	2 oz	176	138	78
cheese (Dairy Queen)	1 serving	330	189	57
chilli (Dairy Queen)	1 serving	320	180	56
regular (Dairy Queen)	1 serving	280	144	51
super (Dairy Queen)	1 serving	520	243	47
Hot five-bean salad ✔	1 cup	293	90	31
Hot fudge brownie delight (Dairy Queen)	1 serving	600	225	38
Hot fudge sundae (McDonald's)	1 sundae	310	85	27
Hot ham 'n cheese (Hardee's)	1 sandwich	330	108	33
Hot mulled cider ✔	1 cup	176	0	0
Hotcakes, with butter and syrup (McDonald's)	1 serving	410	83	20
House salad dressing (Burger King)	1 packet	260	234	90
Huevos rancheros ✔	1 egg	466	25	5
Hummus ✔	1/4 cup	105	47	45
Hush puppies, deep fried, 1 1/2" diameter	1 piece	51	16	31

FOOD

CALORIES

	AMOUNT	TOTAL	FAT	%FAT

I

	AMOUNT	TOTAL	FAT	%FAT
I.M.O., imitation sour cream	1 Tbsp	30	27	90
	1 cup	480	432	90
Ice cream				
(Baskin Robbins)	1 cup	470	236	50
sugar free	1 cup	200	36	18
brick, any flavor	1 cup	295	144	49
bulk (Breyers)	1 cup	300	144	48
(Haagen Dazs)	1 cup	546	306	56
Ice cream cone				
plain, without ice cream	1 cone	18	2	11
sugar, without ice cream	1 cone	49	39	80
waffle, without ice cream	1 average	118	25	21
Ice cream float (Dairy Queen)	1 serving	410	63	15
Ice cream sandwich, 2.5 oz	1 bar	162	45	28
Ice milk				
brick, 4.4 oz	1 cup	185	54	29
Dreyer's Grand Light	1 cup	240	90	38
soft serve, 5.8 oz	1 cup	225	45	20
Imitation mayonnaise	1 Tbsp	50	45	90
Instant Breakfast, with 3.8% milk (Carnation)	1 cup	280	81	29
International coffees, all varieties				
regular	6 oz	55	24	44
sugar free	6 oz	30	18	60
Irish coffee ✔	6 oz	154	81	53
Italian bread, 4 1/2 x 3 1/2 x 1"	1 slice	85	tr	tr
Italian salad dressing				
oil free	1 Tbsp	4	0	0
reduced calorie	1 Tbsp	10	9	90
regular	1 Tbsp	85	80	94
reduced calorie (Burger King)	1 packet	30	18	60

FOOD

CALORIES

	AMOUNT	TOTAL	FAT	%FAT

J

FOOD	AMOUNT	TOTAL	FAT	%FAT
Jalapeno peppers, chopped	1/2 cup	17	tr	tr
Jam and jelly, all varieties				
regular	1 tsp	18	tr	tr
	1 Tbsp	55	tr	tr
1/2 oz packet	1 packet	40	tr	tr
low sugar	1 Tbsp	24	tr	tr
	1 tsp	8	tr	tr
Jam thumbprints ✔	1 cookie	84	45	54
Japanese style vegtables				
in seasoned sauce, frozen	3.3 oz	90	45	50
Jambalaya, shrimp ✔	1 cup	450	153	34
Jarlsberg cheese	1 oz	100	63	63
Jello (Skipper's)	1/2 cup	55	0	0
Jelly beans, 10 pieces = 1 oz	1 oz	101	1	1
2 oz = 1/4 cup	1/4 cup	202	3	1
Jelly roll ✔	1/10 cake	161	27	17
Jerky, beef	1 oz	108	43	40
Jicama, fresh	1/2 cup	48	tr	tr
Just Right (Kellogg's)	1 cup	150	0	0

FOOD

CALORIES

	AMOUNT	TOTAL	FAT	%FAT

K

	AMOUNT	TOTAL	FAT	%FAT
Kahlua, 63 proof	1 oz	107	0	0
Kale, fresh or frozen, cooked	1/2 cup	23	4	17
Kidney beans				
canned	1 cup	135	6	4
cooked	1 cup	218	8	4
dry	1 cup	635	25	4
Kielbasa	1 oz	88	69	79
Kisses (Hershey)	1 kiss	25	14	56
6 kisses = 1 oz	1 oz	150	84	56
Kiwi, fresh, medium	1 kiwi	50	tr	tr
Kix (General Mills)	1 cup	73	6	8
Knockwurst	1 oz	87	71	82
Kohlrabi, fresh, cooked	1/2 cup	18	tr	tr
Kool aid, diluted				
sugar free	8 oz	2	0	0
with sugar	8 oz	90	0	0
Kuchen ✔	1 piece	225	63	28
Kumquat, fresh, medium	1 kumquat	12	tr	tr

L

	AMOUNT	TOTAL	FAT	%FAT
Lamb chop, with bone, broiled	1.7 oz	92	36	39
Lamb, leg of, whole, roasted	1 oz	54	20	37
Lamb shoulder, whole, braised	1 oz	80	41	51

FOOD

CALORIES

	AMOUNT	TOTAL	FAT	%FAT
Lard	1 Tbsp	117	117	100
	1 cup	1849	1849	100
Lasagna noodles, cut				
cooked	1 cup	200	12	6
dry	1 cup	225	13	6
long, dry, 3 noodles = 2 oz	2 oz	210	9	4
Lasagna				
4 x 3 x 2" ✔	1 piece	633	396	63
with meat sauce, frozen (Stouffer's)	21 oz	720	234	33
	10 1/2 oz	360	117	33
Laughing Cow, reduced calorie cheese	1 oz	50	27	54
Le Creme topping	1 Tbsp	12	9	75
	1 cup	192	144	75
Lefse, 10" diameter ✔	1 lefse	79	15	19
Lemon cream pie ✔				
1/6 of 9"	1 piece	327	144	44
1/8 of 9"	1 piece	245	108	44
9", whole	1 pie	1960	864	44
Lemon juice, fresh,				
canned or bottled, unsweetened	1 Tbsp	3	tr	tr
	8 oz	55	tr	tr
Lemon meringue pie ✔				
1/6 of 9"	1 piece	357	129	36
1/8 of 9"	1 piece	268	96	36
9", whole	1 pie	2142	771	36
Lemon, fresh	1 lemon	20	tr	tr
Lemonade, frozen				
concentrate	6 oz	425	tr	tr
reconstituted	8 oz	105	tr	tr
Lentil Soup				
homemade ✔	1 cup	247	45	18
(Progresso)	1 cup	143	29	20
Lentils				
cooked	1 cup	210	tr	tr
dry	1 cup	680	10	1
Less Bread	1 slice	40	tr	tr

FOOD

CALORIES

	AMOUNT	TOTAL	FAT	%FAT
Lettuce				
butterhead, 5" diameter	1 head	25	tr	tr
iceberg, 6" diameter	1 head	70	8	11
pieces	1 cup	5	tr	tr
wedge, 1/4 head	1 wedge	15	tr	tr
romaine, chopped	1 cup	10	2	20
lettuce leaves	1 leaf	tr	tr	tr
Licorice, stick, 0.35 oz	1 average	35	tr	tr
Life Saver	1 average	8	tr	tr
Light N' Lively cheese (Kraft)	1 oz	70	36	51
Lima beans				
canned or frozen	1/2 cup	84	2	2
large, cooked	1 cup	276	11	4
dry	1 cup	690	29	4
small, cooked	1 cup	262	10	4
dry	1 cup	656	27	4
Lima Beans with Ham (Dennison's)	1 cup	267	63	24
Limburger cheese	1 oz	90	66	73
Lime juice, fresh or canned, unsweetened	1 Tbsp	4	tr	tr
	8 oz	65	tr	tr
Lime, fresh	1 lime	28	2	7
Limeade, frozen				
concentrate	6 oz	410	tr	tr
reconstituted	8 oz	100	tr	tr
Linguini with Scallops and Clams, frozen (Buget Gourmet Slim Selects)	9 1/2 oz	280	99	35
Lite Catch Meals (Skipper's)				
3 chicken strips and salad	1 basket	310	135	44
1 fish fillet, 2 chicken strips and salad	1 basket	403	189	47
2 fish fillets and salad	1 basket	413	207	50
Lite-Line, 1 1/2 slice = 1 oz	1 oz	50	18	36
low cholesterol	1 oz	90	63	70
Liver and onions ✔	4 oz liver	318	163	51
Liver pate, chicken	1 Tbsp	69	59	86
Liver sausage	1 oz	97	81	84

FOOD		CALORIES		
	AMOUNT	TOTAL	FAT	%FAT
Liver				
beef, fried	1 oz	65	27	42
calf, fried	1 oz	75	34	45
raw	1 oz	40	12	30
chicken, simmered	1 oz	47	11	23
Liverwurst spread	1 oz	91	69	76
Lobster				
grilled, with butter	5 oz	232	117	50
steamed	1 oz	28	2	7
Loganberries, fresh	1/2 cup	45	4	9
Loquats, fresh	1 whole	6	tr	tr
Lox	1 oz	33	11	33
Lutefisk, raw	1 oz	30	3	10

M

M & M's Peanut Candies	1 oz	143	64	45
	1 lb	2288	1024	45
M & M's Plain Candies	1 oz	142	53	37
	1 lb	2240	864	39
Macadamia nuts, whole, 12 = 1 oz	1 oz	206	199	97
4.8 oz = 1 cup	1 cup	988	955	97
Macaroni and cheese				
(Kraft)	1 cup	363	146	40
canned	1 cup	230	90	39
from mix	1 cup	267	24	9
frozen dinner (Swanson)	12 1/4 oz	380	135	36
with 3.8% milk ✔	1 cup	305	198	65
with skim milk ✔	1 cup	281	171	61

FOOD

CALORIES

	AMOUNT	TOTAL	FAT	%FAT
Macaroni and cheese with Mini-Franks				
frozen (Banquet Kid Cuisine)	9 oz	380	126	33
Macaroni salad, with mayonnaise ✔	1/2 cup	167	53	32
Macaroni, cooked				
firm	1 cup	207	6	3
tender	1 cup	151	5	3
Macaroni, dry	1 cup	405	12	3
Macaroni, spinach				
cooked	1 cup	155	5	3
dry	1 cup	524	15	3
Macaroon cookie, 3" diameter	1 cookie	98	41	42
(Dunkin' Donuts)	1 cookie	351	171	49
Mackerel				
broiled	1 oz	75	46	61
canned	1 oz	51	26	51
Maltballs, carob-coated	1 oz	108	19	18
Malted milk, made with 3.8% milk	8 oz	236	89	38
Malted milkshake (Dairy Queen)	1 small	520	108	21
	1 regular	760	162	21
	1 large	1060	225	21
Mandarin Chicken, frozen (Budget Gourmet)	10 oz	290	54	19
Mandarin oranges, canned, unsweetened	1/2 cup	31	4	13
fresh, 2 3/8" diameter	1 average	37	tr	tr
Mango, fresh, medium	1 mango	152	7	5
Manhattan clam chowder ✔	1 cup	276	90	33
Manhattan cocktail	4 oz	186	0	0
Manicotti Milano, frozen (Stouffer's)	10 oz	360	180	50
Manicotti, large noodle, dry	2 pieces	102	9	9
Manicotti, stuffed ✔	1 each	188	54	29
Manwich, canned, Mexican (Hunt-Wesson)	1/4 cup	32	0	0
Maple bar, or Long John, 5 x 2"	1 piece	324	179	55
Maple syrup				
imitation flavor	1 Tbsp	59	0	0
real	1 Tbsp	50	0	0

FOOD	AMOUNT	CALORIES		
		TOTAL	FAT	%FAT
Margarine				
diet	1 tsp	17	17	100
	1 Tbsp	50	50	100
	1 cup	815	815	100
soft, tub, regular	1 tsp	34	34	100
	1 Tbsp	102	102	100
	1 cup	1634	1634	100
stick, regular	1 tsp	34	34	100
	1 pat	36	36	100
	1 Tbsp	102	102	100
	1 cup	1634	1634	100
whipped, "lite"	1 tsp	23	23	100
	1 Tbsp	68	68	100
	1 cup	1087	1087	100
Marshmallow cookie, with coconut or chocolate topping	1 cookie	74	22	30
Marshmallow Creme, topping (Kraft)	1 Tbsp	45	0	0
Marshmallows, 1 x 1 x 1"	1 piece	18	tr	tr
Martini cocktail	4 oz	160	0	0
Mashed potatoes				
homemade ✔	1/2 cup	81	20	25
with gravy (Kentucky Fried Chicken)	1 serving	71	14	20
Matzo ball, 2" diameter	1 ball	123	74	60
Matzoh cracker	1 piece	117	3	3
Maximelt (Taco Bell)	1 serving	266	139	52
Mayonnaise	1 tsp	33	33	100
	1 Tbsp	100	99	99
Light (Kraft)	1 Tbsp	45	45	100
reduced calorie				
(Heart Beat)	1 Tbsp	40	36	90
(Weight Watchers)	1 Tbsp	50	45	90
(Saffola)	1 Tbsp	100	99	99
McChicken sandwich (McDonald's)	1 sandwich	490	257	53
McDLT sandwich (McDonald's)	1 burger	580	331	57
McDonaldland cookies (McDonald's)	1 box	290	83	29

FOOD

CALORIES

	AMOUNT	TOTAL	FAT	%FAT
McMuffin (McDonald's)				
sausage	1 serving	370	197	53
sausage with egg	1 serving	440	241	55
Measure Up Bread	1 slice	40	18	45
Meat Loaf ✔				
1 1/2 x 4 x 2"	1 slice	417	243	58
all beef	1 oz	51	20	39
with beef and pork	1 oz	53	22	42
Meat Loaf dinner, frozen (Swanson)	10 3/4 oz	430	198	46
Meatballs with tomato sauce ✔	1 cup	209	136	65
Meat, canned, potted	1 Tbsp	30	18	60
Melba toast, plain	1 slice	15	2	13
Melon balls, cantaloupe or				
honeydew, frozen	1/2 cup	72	2	3
Mexican Style Combination dinner, frozen				
(Swanson)	14 1/4 oz	520	216	42
Mexican pizza (Taco Bell)	1 serving	575	331	58
Milk				
1%	8 oz	102	24	24
2%, lowfat	8 oz	122	42	34
3.8%, whole	8 oz	161	81	50
chocolate				
1%	8 oz	160	26	16
2%, lowfat	8 oz	180	45	25
3.8%, whole	8 oz	210	72	34
instant nonfat dry	1 cup	245	tr	tr
reconstituted	8 oz	81	tr	tr
skim	8 oz	85	tr	tr
Milk, condensed, sweetened	8 oz	980	243	25
Milk, evaporated, unsweetened				
skim	8 oz	200	9	5
whole	8 oz	340	171	50
Milk, goat	8 oz	163	88	54
Milkshake				
chocolate (Burger King)	1 shake	320	108	34
chocolate (Hardee's)	1 shake	460	72	16

FOOD

CALORIES

	AMOUNT	TOTAL	FAT	%FAT
Milkshake (continued)				
chocolate (McDonald's)	1 shake	390	95	24
Jamocha (Arby's)	1 shake	368	95	26
large (Dairy Queen)	1 shake	990	234	24
regular (Dairy Queen)	1 shake	710	171	24
small (Dairy Queen)	1 shake	490	117	24
strawberry (McDonald's)	1 shake	380	91	24
vanilla (Burger King)	1 shake	321	90	28
vanilla (McDonald's)	1 shake	350	92	26
Milky Way, regular size, 2 oz	1 bar	260	81	31
snack size, 0.8 oz	1 bar	100	36	36
Millet				
cooked	1 cup	165	13	8
dry	1 cup	660	53	8
Mincemeat pie, double crust ✔				
1/6 of 9"	1 piece	672	352	52
1/8 of 9"	1 piece	504	264	52
9", whole	1 pie	4032	2112	52
Mineral water	8 oz	0	0	0
Mineral water and juice soda	10 oz	124	0	0
Minestrone soup				
homemade ✔	1 cup	79	15	19
(Progresso)	1 cup	134	22	16
with water (Campbell's)	1 cup	71	18	25
Miracle Whip				
Light (Kraft)	1 Tbsp	45	36	80
regular (Kraft)	1 Tbsp	68	62	91
Mixed fruit, dried	1 oz	73	1	1
Mixed vegetables, canned	1/2 cup	35	tr	tr
Mocha Mix, non-dairy dessert				
chocolate, mocha or almond	1 cup	300	162	54
vanilla or strawberry	1 cup	280	126	45
Molasses				
dark, blackstrap	1 Tbsp	45	tr	tr
light	1 Tbsp	50	tr	tr
sorghum	1 Tbsp	55	tr	tr

FOOD   CALORIES

	AMOUNT	TOTAL	FAT	%FAT
Molly McButter, all flavors	1 tsp	8	0	0
Monterey Jack cheese	1 oz	106	76	72
Light Naturals (Kraft)	1 oz	80	45	56
Moo goo gai pan ✔	1 cup	566	307	54
Mounds, 1.90 oz	1 bar	260	126	48
Mousse ✔				
chocolate	1/2 cup	246	191	78
strawberry	1/2 cup	248	195	79
Mozzarella cheese				
Light Naturals (Kraft)	1 oz	80	36	45
part skim	1 oz	72	40	56
whole milk	1 oz	90	62	69
Mozzarella, low moisture, part skim	1 oz	78	43	55
Mr. Misty (Dairy Queen)				
float	1 serving	390	63	16
freeze	1 serving	500	108	22
kiss	1 serving	70	0	0
Muenster cheese	1 oz	104	75	72
Mueslix, Bran (Kellogg's)	1 cup	280	36	13
Muffin, 3" diameter				
blueberry	1 muffin	298	172	58
bran with raisins	1 muffin	271	58	21
corn	1 muffin	215	92	43
oat bran	1 muffin	290	86	30
pumpkin with raisins	1 muffin	287	97	34
Muffin, 4" diameter				
blueberry	1 muffin	397	229	58
bran with raisins	1 muffin	361	77	21
corn	1 muffin	287	122	43
oat bran	1 muffin	387	115	30
pumpkin with raisins	1 muffin	382	130	34
Muffins (Dunkin' Donuts)				
apple spice	1 muffin	327	99	30
banana nut	1 muffin	327	108	33
blueberry	1 muffin	263	90	34
bran	1 muffin	353	117	33

FOOD

CALORIES

	AMOUNT	TOTAL	FAT	%FAT
Muffins (Dunkin' Donuts continued)				
cherry	1 muffin	317	90	28
corn	1 muffin	347	117	34
Mung bean sprouts, raw	1 cup	37	2	5
Mung beans				
cooked	1 cup	355	12	3
dry	1 cup	714	24	3
Mushroom 'n Swiss burger (Hardee's)	1 burger	490	243	50
Mushrooms				
canned, drained	1/2 cup	26	5	19
raw, sliced	1/2 cup	10	tr	tr
Muskmellon, fresh, 5" diameter	1/2 melon	82	3	4
Mussels, steamed	1 oz	49	12	24
Mustard greens	1/2 cup	15	4	27
Mustard				
dry	1 tsp	12	8	67
with horseradish	1 tsp	4	2	50
yellow	1 tsp	5	tr	tr
My Meatballs and Shells				
frozen (My Own Meals)	8 oz	210	81	39

N

	AMOUNT	TOTAL	FAT	%FAT
Nachos (Taco Bell)	1 serving	346	167	48
Bellgrande	1 serving	649	318	49
Navy or pea beans				
cooked	1 cup	224	10	4
dry	1 cup	697	30	4
Nectarine, fresh, 2 1/2" diameter	1 fruit	88	tr	tr

FOOD

CALORIES

	AMOUNT	TOTAL	FAT	%FAT
Neufchatel, reduced fat cream cheese	1 oz	74	58	78
New England clam chowder ✔	1 cup	327	126	39
(Progresso)	1 cup	185	94	51
Noodles				
chow mein, canned	1 cup	220	108	49
egg, cooked	1 cup	200	21	11
egg, dry	1 cup	283	30	11
plain, cooked	1 cup	146	4	3
plain, dry	1 cup	248	7	3
spinach, cooked	1 cup	200	22	11
Norwegian flat bread (Kavli)	1 wafer	35	0	0
Nutri-Grain Almond Raisin (Kellogg's)	1 cup	186	24	13
Nutri-Grain Wheat (Kellogg's)	1 cup	165	0	0

O

	AMOUNT	TOTAL	FAT	%FAT
Oat bran bread, 4 1/4 x 5 x 3/4"	1 slice	84	9	11
Oat Bran Flakes (Kellogg's)	1 cup	200	14	7
Oat bran muffin				
3" diameter	1 muffin	290	86	30
4" diameter	1 muffin	387	115	30
Oat Bran Options (Ralston)	1 cup	130	9	7
Oat nut bread, 4 x 5 x 1/2"	1 slice	100	18	18
Oatmeal cookie				
homemade ✔	1 cookie	80	29	36
Big Batch mix	1 cookie	130	54	42
36 cookies	1 pkg	4680	1944	42
with raisins, 3" diameter	1 cookie	82	25	30

FOOD		CALORIES		
	AMOUNT	TOTAL	FAT	%FAT
Oatmeal, quick or old fashioned				
cooked	1 cup	148	25	17
dry	1 cup	333	57	17
Oatmeal, instant, cooked, 1 packet				
apples and cinnamon	3/4 cup	120	9	8
maple and brown sugar	3/4 cup	150	18	12
raisin, date and walnut	3/4 cup	140	36	26
regular	3/4 cup	90	18	20
Oats, rolled				
cooked	1 cup	148	25	17
dry	1 cup	333	57	17
Octopus, raw	1 oz	21	2	10
Oil and vinegar salad dressing, regular (Kraft)	1 Tbsp	70	63	90
Oil, salad or cooking, all types	1 tsp	40	40	100
	1 Tbsp	120	120	100
	1 cup	1927	1927	100
Okra pods, 3 x 5/8"	10 pods	30	tr	tr
Old Fashioned cocktail	6 oz	269	0	0
Olives				
black, ripe, extra large	1 olive	9	8	89
sliced	1 cup	174	155	89
Greek	1 olive	7	6	86
green, large, 1" diameter	1 olive	5	4	80
small	1 olive	3	3	100
Omelet (Wendy's)				
cheese	1 omelet	290	189	65
cheese, mushroom	1 omelet	250	153	61
ham, cheese, green pepper, onion	1 omelet	280	171	61
mushroom, green pepper, onion	1 omelet	210	135	64
Omelet, French, 2 eggs ✔	2 eggs	266	207	78
Onion				
dehydrated flakes	1 Tbsp	13	tr	tr
fresh, cooked	1/2 cup	30	tr	tr
raw, 2 1/4" diameter	1 onion	38	1	3
chopped	1/2 cup	33	tr	tr
sliced	1/2 cup	23	tr	tr

FOOD

CALORIES

	AMOUNT	TOTAL	FAT	%FAT
Onion dip ✔	1 Tbsp	55	54	98
Onion rings				
homemade ✔	10 rings	352	207	59
french fried (Burger King)	1 serving	274	144	53
french fried, 3 oz = 1 serving	1 serving	285	140	49
Onion soup	1 cup	35	8	23
dehydrated, 1.5 oz	1 pkg	150	45	30
Onions with cream sauce, frozen	5 oz	140	90	64
Orange Drink (Hi-C)	8 oz	136	0	0
Orange juice				
canned or frozen, reconstituted				
unsweetened	8 oz	120	tr	tr
dehydrated crystals, reconstituted	8 oz	115	tr	tr
frozen, concentrate	6 oz	360	tr	tr
Orange/grapefruit juice				
frozen concentrate	6 oz	330	8	2
reconstituted	8 oz	110	tr	tr
Orange, fresh, 3" diameter	1 orange	73	tr	tr
sections	1/2 cup	45	tr	tr
Oreo cookie (Nabisco)	1 cookie	40	18	45
Oriental Beef with Vegetable and Rice, frozen (Lean Cuisine)	8 5/8 oz	250	63	25
Oriental Beef, frozen (Budget Gourmet Slim Selects)	10 oz	290	81	28
Oriental noodles, Ramen, 3 oz = 1 pkg	1 pkg	390	153	39
Oriental party mix	1 oz	150	81	54
Oriental style vegetables, frozen	3.3 oz	30	0	0
Orzo, cooked	1 cup	210	9	4
dry	1 cup	630	27	4
Ovaltine, malt or chocolate powder	3/4 oz	78	8	10
Oven browned potatoes ✔	1 cup	211	45	21
Oyster crackers	10 cracker	43	10	23
Oyster stew ✔	1 cup	233	138	59

FOOD	AMOUNT	CALORIES		
		TOTAL	FAT	%FAT
Oysters				
breaded, fried, large, 1 oz	1 whole	56	32	57
Pacific, raw	1 oz	26	5	19
	1 cup	218	48	22
large	1 whole	52	11	21
medium	1 whole	38	8	21
small	1 whole	24	5	21
steamed	1 oz	39	13	33
Oysters Rockefeller ✔	6 oysters	200	99	50

P

FOOD	AMOUNT	TOTAL	FAT	%FAT
Pancake syrup				
fruit flavored	1 Tbsp	59	0	0
maple flavored	1 Tbsp	59	0	0
reduced sugar, "lite"	1 Tbsp	30	0	0
Pancake				
4" diameter ✔	1 pancake	104	29	28
from "complete" mix, 4" diameter	1 pancake	70	27	39
from mix				
4" diameter	1 pancake	122	36	30
6" diameter	1 pancake	164	48	29
blueberry, 4" diameter	1 pancake	134	27	20
buckwheat, 4" diameter	1 pancake	108	46	43
buckwheat, 6" diameter	1 pancake	146	59	40
Papaya, fresh				
1/2" cubes	1/2 cup	28	tr	tr
3 1/2" diameter	1 papaya	119	2	2

FOOD

CALORIES

	AMOUNT	TOTAL	FAT	%FAT
Parfait (Dairy Queen)	1 serving	430	72	17
double delight (Dairy Queen)	1 serving	490	180	37
peanut buster (Dairy Queen)	1 serving	740	306	41
Parmesan cheese, grated	1 Tbsp	25	18	72
	1 oz	120	86	72
	1/2 cup	200	144	72
Parsley	1 Tbsp	tr	tr	tr
Parsnips, fresh cooked	1/2 cup	50	4	8
Pasta Carbonara, frozen (Stouffer's)	7 3/4 oz	620	405	65
Pasta Primavera, frozen (Weight Watchers)	8 1/4 oz	290	117	40
Pasta salad with vegetables ✔	1/2 cup	100	51	51
Pastrami	1 oz	106	78	74
Patty melt sandwich on rye	1 sandwich	636	383	60
Pea pods, sugar or snow peas	1/2 cup	26	1	4
Pea salad with cheese ✔	1/2 cup	218	148	68
Peach pie, double crust ✔				
1/6 of 9"	1 piece	402	152	38
1/8 of 9"	1 piece	301	113	38
9", whole	1 pie	2410	910	38
Peaches, canned				
heavy syrup	2 halves	78	1	1
sliced	1/2 cup	78	1	1
juice pack	2 halves	45	1	2
water pack	2 halves	31	1	3
sliced	1/2 cup	31	1	3
Peaches				
dried	1/2 cup	210	4	2
fresh, 2 1/2" diameter	1 peach	40	tr	tr
sliced	1/2 cup	32	1	3
frozen, sliced, sweetened	1/2 cup	110	tr	tr
Peanut brittle	1 oz	120	27	23
Peanut butter cookie, 3" diameter ✔	1 cookie	91	45	49
Peanut Butter Cup (Reese's)	1 average	86	47	55
Peanut Butter 'n Cheese (Handi-Snacks)	1 package	190	117	62
Peanut butter oatmeal bars ✔	1 bar	116	54	47

FOOD

CALORIES

	AMOUNT	TOTAL	FAT	%FAT
Peanut butter sandwich cookie, 1 3/4" diameter	1 cookie	58	21	36
Peanut butter, crunchy or smooth	1 Tbsp	95	72	76
	1 cup	1520	1152	76
Peanuts				
chopped	1 Tbsp	52	40	77
dry roasted	1 oz	174	122	70
5 oz = 1 cup	1 cup	868	612	71
roasted in shell, jumbo size	1 nut	11	8	73
Virginia or Spanish, 45 = 1 oz	1 oz	169	129	76
5 oz = 1 cup	1 cup	844	644	76
whole, without shell	1 oz	140	73	52
5.4 oz = 1 cup	1 cup	756	394	52
Peanut candies				
carob coated	1 oz	140	73	52
yogurt coated	1 oz	129	78	60
Pears, canned				
heavy syrup	2 halves	76	2	3
water pack	2 halves	58	2	3
Pears, fresh, D'Anjou, 3" diameter	1 pear	120	8	7
Peas and carrots, frozen	3.3 oz	60	0	0
Peas with cream sauce, frozen	5 oz	180	99	55
Peas, green				
crowder, shelled	1/2 cup	50	9	18
canned, fresh or frozen, cooked	1/2 cup	68	3	4
raw, shelled	1/2 cup	56	2	4
Peas, split				
cooked	1 cup	230	5	2
dry	1 cup	696	18	3
Peas, whole				
cooked	1 cup	338	11	3
dry	1 cup	680	23	3
Pecan pie, single crust ✔				
1/6 of 9"	1 piece	575	283	49
1/8 of 9"	1 piece	431	212	49
9", whole	1 pie	3449	1700	49

FOOD

CALORIES

	AMOUNT	TOTAL	FAT	%FAT
Pecan pie, snack size (Sara Lee)	1 pie	260	117	45
Pecans, halves				
20 = 1 oz	1 oz	195	182	93
3.8 oz = 1 cup	1 cup	742	693	93
Pectin				
Certo, liquid	1/2 cup	12	0	0
Sure-Jell, dry	1 oz	76	0	0
Pepper Steak with Rice, frozen				
(Budget Gourmet)	10 oz	300	81	27
Pepper, bell, green or red	1 large	22	2	9
Pepper, stuffed, 2 3/4" long ✔	1 pepper	322	167	52
Peppercorn salad dressing (McDonald's)	1 packet	400	392	98
Peppermint patty, chocolate covered	1 oz	116	27	23
Pepperoni	1 oz	141	112	79
Peppers, hot, chili (Old El Paso)	1 Tbsp	4	0	0
Pepsi Cola	12 oz	156	0	0
Pepsi Light	12 oz	1	0	0
Perch, broiled	1 oz	33	3	9
Persimmon, fresh	1 fruit	103	2	2
Pesto, basil ✔	1 Tbsp	123	117	95
Pheasant, raw	1 oz	43	13	30
Philly steak sandwich, 3 oz meat	1 sandwich	402	162	40
Philly Swiss burger (Wendy's)	1 burger	510	216	42
Pickle relish				
sour	1 Tbsp	3	tr	tr
sweet	1 Tbsp	20	tr	tr
Pickled beets, canned	1/2 cup	55	tr	tr
Pickles				
dill, medium, whole	1 pickle	5	tr	tr
sweet gherkins, whole	1 pickle	20	tr	tr
Pico de Gallo (Taco Bell)	1 serving	8	2	25
Piecrust, double crust ✔				
1/6 of 9"	1/6 crust	300	176	59
1/8 of 9"	1/8 crust	226	132	58
9", whole	2 crusts	1800	1056	59

FOOD | CALORIES

	AMOUNT	TOTAL	FAT	%FAT
Piecrust, mix, double crust				
9", 10 oz pkg	1 pkg	1485	818	55
Piecrust, single crust ✔				
1/6 of 9"	1 piece	150	88	59
1/8 of 9"	1 piece	113	66	58
9", whole	1 crust	900	528	59
Pierogies, 1 3/4 x 1 3/4" ✔	1 piece	75	35	47
Pimiento cheese, processed	1 oz	106	80	75
Pine nuts or pinon nuts	1 oz	156	104	67
2.5 oz = 1 cup	1 cup	388	260	67
Pineapple, canned				
chunks, juice pack	1/2 cup	40	tr	tr
crushed, in syrup	1/2 cup	95	tr	tr
slices, in heavy syrup	1 slice	74	1	1
tibits, water pack	1/2 cup	48	tr	tr
Pineapple, dried	1 oz	74	3	4
Pineapple, fresh, diced	1/2 cup	40	tr	tr
Pineapple juice				
canned, unsweetened	8 oz	138	tr	tr
frozen, concentrate	6 oz	387	3	1
reconstituted	8 oz	130	1	1
Pineapple upside down cake				
1/9 of 8" square	1 piece	270	90	33
8" square	1 cake	2430	810	33
Pinto or calico beans				
cooked	1 cup	288	9	3
dry	1 cup	663	20	3
Pintos and cheese (Taco Bell)	1 serving	190	78	41
Pistachio nuts, with shell				
4.4 oz = 1 cup	1 cup	748	607	81
50 = 1 oz	1 oz	170	138	81
Pita/pocket bread, white or whole wheat	1 bread	163	7	4
Pizza, deep dish, cheese/tomato,				
5 1/4 x 3 3/4"	1 slice	421	122	29

FOOD		CALORIES		
	AMOUNT	TOTAL	FAT	%FAT
Pizza, 1/8 of 16" diameter (Domino's)				
cheese	1 slice	188	45	24
deluxe	1 slice	249	92	37
double cheese, pepperoni	1 slice	273	114	42
ham, Canadian-style	1 slice	209	50	24
pepperoni	1 slice	230	79	34
sausage, mushroom	1 slice	215	71	33
veggie	1 slice	249	83	34
Pizza, pan, 18 of 14" diameter, medium (Pizza Hut)				
cheese	1 slice	246	81	33
pepperoni	1 slice	270	99	37
supreme	1 slice	295	135	46
super supreme	1 slice	282	117	41
Pizza, personal pan, 4 1/2" diameter (Pizza Hut)				
pepperoni	1 pizza	338	131	39
supreme	1 pizza	324	126	39
Pizza, Thin 'n Crispy, 15" (Pizza Hut)				
cheese	1 pizza	1592	616	38
pepperoni	1 pizza	1656	720	43
supreme	1 pizza	1840	792	43
super supreme	1 pizza	1856	760	41
Pizza, Thin 'n Crispy 1/8 of 15", medium (Pizza Hut)				
cheese	1 slice	199	77	38
pepperoni	1 slice	207	90	43
supreme	1 slice	230	99	43
super supreme	1 slice	232	95	41
Pizza, 12" diameter, frozen				
Canadian bacon, thin crust	1 pizza	1449	423	29
double topping, no meat	1 pizza	2402	891	37
with meat	1 pizza	2483	1017	41
sausage, pepperoni or hamburger thin crust	1 pizza	1507	486	32

FOOD

CALORIES

	AMOUNT	TOTAL	FAT	%FAT
Pizza, 1/8 of 12" diameter, frozen				
Canadian bacon, thin crust	1 slice	181	53	29
double topping, no meat	1 slice	301	111	37
with meat	1 slice	310	127	41
sausage, pepperoni or hamburger				
thin crust	1 slIce	188	61	32
Pizza, Mexican (Taco Bell)	1 serving	575	331	58
Plantain	I fruit	119	4	3
Plums, canned				
heavy syrup	3 plums	83	1	1
water pack	3 plums	44	1	2
Plums, fresh				
1 1/2" diameter	1 plum	20	tr	tr
2 1/8" diameter	1 plum	30	tr	tr
Polenta ✔	1/3 cup	72	9	13
Polish sausage				
10" x 1 1/4"	8 oz	690	516	75
5 3/8" x 1"	2.7 oz	231	172	74
Pollack, Walleye, broiled	1 oz	32	3	9
Pomegranate, pulp only, 2 3/8 x 3/8"	1 fruit	97	4	4
Popcorn				
air popped, unbuttered	1 cup	25	2	8
microwave, pouch type	1 cup	35	18	51
caramel	1 cup	96	50	52
cheddar cheese	1 cup	50	30	60
light	1 cup	17	3	18
oil popped, buttered with 2 tsp	1 cup	108	86	80
unbuttered	1 cup	40	18	45
unpopped	1 cup	742	84	11
Popover ✔	1 average	112	41	37
Popsicle				
(Crystal Light)	1 average	13	tr	tr
(Jell-O)	1 average	30	tr	tr
Pork and beans	1 cup	237	18	8

FOOD

CALORIES

	AMOUNT	TOTAL	FAT	%FAT
Pork chop, sirloin, broiled	1 oz	69	34	49
center loin, broiled	1 oz	65	27	42
top loin, broiled	1 oz	73	38	52
Pork chow mein, with rice ✔	1 1/2 cups	464	234	50
Pork feet, simmered	1 oz	55	31	56
Pork links, cooked	1oz	110	81	74
Pork sausage, cooked				
(Brown and Serve)	1 oz	118	95	81
regular	1/2 cup	280	211	75
Pork, shoulder, whole, roasted	1 oz	69	38	55
Pork, shoulder, Boston blade, roasted	1 oz	73	43	59
Port du Salut cheese	1 oz	100	72	72
Post Toasties (Post)	1 cup	80	tr	tr
Postum, instant, powder	2 Tbsp	36	tr	tr
Pot cheese	1 oz	25	tr	tr
Pot pie, beef, 4 1/4" diameter ✔	1 pie	558	296	53
Pot Pie, frozen (Swanson)				
beef	7 oz	380	180	47
chicken	7 oz	380	198	52
turkey	7 oz	380	198	52
Pot roast, beef, cooked	1 oz	65	25	38
Potato				
baked, with skin, 5 x 2", medium	1 potato	145	2	1
boiled, without skin, diced	1/2 cup	51	1	2
Potato Bread ✔	1 slice	92	9	10
Potato Buds, instant, dry flakes	1/3 cup	60	0	0
reconstituted, with fat and milk	1/2 cup	130	54	42
Potato cakes, 3 oz (Arby's)	1 serving	204	108	53
Potato chips				
45 = 1 1/8 oz (Frito Lay)	1 1/8 oz	170	99	58
Bar-B-Que (Frito Lay)	1 oz	150	81	54
O'Grady, 1 oz (Frito Lay)	8 chips	150	81	54
(Pringle's)	1 oz	170	117	69
Ruffles, 25 = 1 1/8 oz (Frito Lay)	1 1/8 oz	170	90	53
Sour Cream and Onion (Frito Lay)	1 oz	160	90	56
Potato pancakes, 8" diameter ✔	1 pancake	495	113	23

FOOD		CALORIES		
	AMOUNT	TOTAL	FAT	%FAT
Potato salad ✔				
hot, German	1/2 cup	139	48	35
with eggs and mayonnaise	1/2 cup	181	92	51
Potato, baked, 9 oz (Wendy's)				
plain	1 large	250	18	7
with bacon and cheese	1 large	570	270	47
with broccoli and cheese	1 large	500	225	45
with cheese	1 large	590	306	52
with chili and cheese	1 large	510	180	35
with sour cream and chives	1 large	460	216	47
Potato-ham scallop ✔	1 1/4 cups	540	207	38
Potatoes				
au gratin ✔	1/2 cup	177	90	51
hashbrowned	1/2 cup	177	81	46
mashed, homemade ✔	1/2 cup	81	20	25
instant, with fat and milk	1/2 cup	96	32	33
scalloped, without cheese ✔	1/2 cup	127	45	35
Potatoes, breakfast, 3 oz (Wendy's)	1 serving	360	198	55
Poulsbo bread, 4 1/2 x 4 x 1/2"	1 slice	105	14	13
Poultry skin, baked	1 oz	122	91	75
Pound cake				
1/12 of loaf	1 slice	160	84	53
8 1/2 x 3 1/2 x 3 1/4"	1 loaf	1920	1008	53
snack size (Sara Lee)	1 cake	200	99	50
Prawns, raw	1 oz	23	1	4
Pretzels				
Dutch, 28 per lb	1 large	58	2	3
soft	1 pretzel	158	27	17
three ring, 148 per lb	1 piece	12	1	8
very thin sticks, 1600 per lb	1 piece	10	tr	tr
Product 19 (Kellogg's)	1 cup	100	0	0
Provolone cheese	1 oz	100	70	70
Prune juice, canned or bottled	8 oz	195	tr	tr
Prunes, dried				
cooked, unsweetened	1/2 cup	128	4	3
large	1 prune	25	0	0

FOOD		CALORIES		
	AMOUNT	TOTAL	FAT	%FAT
Pudding Pops (Jell-O)	1 average	75	18	24
Pudding, all flavors				
with 1% milk (Jell-O)	1/2 cup	140	12	9
with 2% milk (Jell-O)	1/2 cup	150	21	14
with skim milk (Jell-O)	1/2 cup	133	0	0
Pudding, bread, with raisins ✔	1/2 cup	209	60	29
Pudding, instant mix				
with 1% milk (Jell-O)	1/2 cup	150	12	8
with 2% milk (Jell-O)	1/2 cup	160	21	13
with 3.8% milk (Jell-O)	1/2 cup	180	36	20
with skim milk (Jell-O)	1/2 cup	143	0	0
sugar free, with 2% milk	1/2 cup	90	18	20
Pudding, mix				
with skim milk (D-Zerta)	1/2 cup	70	0	0
with 3.8% milk (Jell-O)	1/2 cup	170	36	21
Pudding, rice				
with 2% milk (Jell-O)	1/2 cup	160	30	19
with raisins ✔	1/2 cup	160	31	19
with skim milk (Jell-O)	1/2 cup	143	9	6
Pudding, tapioca				
with 2% milk (Jell-O)	1/2 cup	160	30	19
with 3.8% milk ✔	1/2 cup	110	35	32
with skim milk (Jell-O)	1/2 cup	133	9	7
Puffed Rice (Quaker)	1 cup	51	1	2
Puffed Wheat (Quaker)	1 cup	53	2	4
Pumpernickel bread, 5 x 4 x 3/8"	1 slice	80	tr	tr
Pumpkin bread, 5 x 4 1/2 x 1/2" ✔	1/18 loaf	168	56	33
9 x 5 x 4 1/2"	1 loaf	3032	1014	33
Pumpkin muffin with raisins				
3" diameter	1 muffin	287	97	34
4" diameter	1 muffin	382	130	34
Pumpkin or squash seeds				
138 = 1 oz	1 oz	115	87	76
5.4 oz = 1 cup	1 cup	620	472	76

FOOD

CALORIES

	AMOUNT	TOTAL	FAT	%FAT
Pumpkin pie, single crust ✔				
1/6 of 9"	1 piece	320	153	48
1/8 of 9"	1 piece	240	115	48
9", whole	1 pie	1920	920	48
Pumpkin, fresh cooked or canned	1/2 cup	40	4	10

Q

	AMOUNT	TOTAL	FAT	%FAT
Quarter Pounder (McDonald's)	1 burger	410	186	45
with cheese (McDonald's)	1 burger	520	263	51
Quesadilla ✔	5 oz	739	429	58
Quiche Lorraine, 1/6 of 9" pie ✔	1 piece	543	351	65
Quiche, seafood, 1/6 of 9" pie ✔	1 piece	496	297	60
Quince	1 average	53	1	2

R

	AMOUNT	TOTAL	FAT	%FAT
Rabbit, domestic, stewed	1 oz	61	27	44
Radishes	4 radishes	5	tr	tr
Raisin Bran (Kellogg's)	1 cup	150	11	7

FOOD

CALORIES

	AMOUNT	TOTAL	FAT	%FAT
Raisin bread, 4 x 3 1/2 x 1/2"	1 slice	65	8	12
Raisin Squares (Kellogg's)	1 cup	180	0	0
Raisins				
chocolate coated	1 oz	120	36	30
seedless	1 Tbsp	29	tr	tr
1/2 oz packet	1 packet	40	tr	tr
2.6 oz = 1/2 cup	1/2 cup	210	tr	tr
yogurt coated	1 oz	120	36	30
Ramen oriental noodles, with broth, 3 oz = 1 pkg	1 pkg	390	153	39
Ranch salad dressing (McDonald's)	1 packet	330	310	94
regular (Hidden Valley)	1 Tbsp	54	50	93
reduced calorie	1 Tbsp	40	36	90
Raspberries, black, fresh or canned, unsweetened	1/2 cup	59	9	15
Raspberries, red				
fresh or canned, unsweetened	1/2 cup	43	1	2
frozen, sweetened	1/2 cup	123	2	2
Ravioli				
canned	1 cup	256	72	28
homemade, with meat filling ✔	1 cup	323	113	35
Raw vegetable antipasto ✔	1 cup	355	297	84
Red snapper, broiled	1 oz	36	4	11
Reese's Pieces	1 oz	141	51	36
Refried beans, plain or spicy	1 cup	248	16	6
vegetarian	1 cup	225	34	15
Rhubarb pie, double crust ✔				
1/6 of 9"	1 piece	399	152	38
1/8 of 9"	1 piece	299	113	38
9", whole	1 pie	2391	910	38
Rhubarb, cooked				
unsweetened	1/2 cup	32	tr	tr
sweetened, with 3 Tbsp sugar	1/2 cup	188	tr	tr
Rhubarb, raw, cubed	1 cup	16	tr	tr

FOOD		CALORIES		
	AMOUNT	TOTAL	FAT	%FAT
Rice cakes	1 cake	35	3	9
mini	1 cake	12	tr	tr
Rice Chex (Ralston)	1 cup	96	0	0
Rice Krispies (Kellogg's)	1 cup	110	0	0
Rice noodles, cooked	1 cup	241	36	15
Rice pilaf ✔	1 cup	168	52	31
Rice vinegar				
regular (Marukan)	1 Tbsp	1	0	0
seasoned (Marukan)	1 Tbsp	30	0	0
Rice, brown, instant, cooked	1 cup	240	18	8
Rice, brown, long-grain				
cooked	1 cup	232	14	6
dry	1 cup	666	39	6
Rice, brown, short-grain				
cooked	1 cup	240	11	5
dry	1 cup	720	33	5
Rice, brown, whole grain, fast cooking				
cooked	1 cup	180	18	10
Rice, long grain and wild blend, cooked	1 cup	194	2	1
Rice, white, converted, cooked	1 cup	182	2	1
Rice, white, long-grain				
cooked	1 cup	223	2	1
dry	1 cup	672	6	1
quick, cooked	1 cup	158	2	1
Rice, white, short-grain				
cooked	1 cup	275	2	1
dry	1 cup	726	7	1
Rice, wild				
cooked	1 cup	141	3	2
dry	1 cup	396	7	2
Rice, with red wheat, barley,				
cooked (Hain)	1 cup	180	18	10
Rice-A-Roni				
beef	1/2 cup	110	9	8
chicken	1/2 cup	140	9	6
Spanish	1/2 cup	150	36	24

FOOD	AMOUNT	CALORIES		
		TOTAL	FAT	%FAT
Ricotta cheese				
part skim	1/2 cup	170	84	49
whole milk	1/2 cup	215	141	66
Ricotta, whey, low-fat (Piazza)	1/2 cup	120	36	30
Rigatoni				
cooked	1 cup	100	6	6
dry	1 cup	200	12	6
Ritz cracker	1 cracker	18	8	44
Roast beef sandwich				
hot, with 3 Tbsp gravy	1 sandwich	429	220	51
regular (Arby's)	1 sandwich	353	133	38
super (Arby's)	1 large	501	199	40
big (Hardee's)	1 sandwich	300	99	33
regular (Hardee's)	1 sandwich	260	81	31
Rockfish, broiled	1 oz	35	5	14
Roll, hard, 3 3/4" diameter	1 roll	156	9	6
Roll, onion, 4" diameter	1 roll	190	18	9
Roll, soft				
2" square or cloverleaf	1 roll	83	14	17
dinner ✔	1 roll	98	27	28
(Kentucky Fried Chicken)	1 roll	61	8	13
whole wheat	1 average	90	9	10
Rolled wheat				
cooked	1 cup	180	8	4
dry	1 cup	405	18	4
Rolo caramels	1 oz	140	56	40
Romano cheese, grated	1 Tbsp	19	11	58
	1 oz	114	66	58
	1/2 cup	152	88	58
Root beer	12 oz	150	0	0
sugar free	12 oz	1	0	0
Roquefort cheese	1 oz	105	78	74
Rosettes, 2 1/2" diameter ✔	1 average	33	14	42
Rotini, spirals				
cooked	1 cup	100	9	9
dry	1 cup	200	18	9

FOOD

CALORIES

	AMOUNT	TOTAL	FAT	%FAT
Ruben sandwich on rye	1 sandwich	534	267	50
Rum, 86 proof	1 oz	74	0	0
Russian salad dressing				
reduced calorie	1 Tbsp	27	17	63
regular	1 Tbsp	74	68	92
Rutabaga, fresh cooked, cubed	1/2 cup	35	1	3
Ry-Krisp cracker, natural	1 triple	22	1	5
Rye bread, 4 3/4 x 3 3/4 x 7/16"	1 slice	60	tr	tr
Rye wafers, whole grain	1 wafer	23	tr	tr

S

	AMOUNT	TOTAL	FAT	%FAT
Salami	1 oz	111	84	76
Light and Lean (Hormel)	3/4 oz	40	27	68
Genoa	1 oz	110	90	82
hard	1 oz	115	86	75
Sallisbury Steak ✔	5 oz	596	378	63
Sallisbury Steak dinner, frozen (Swanson)	10 3/4 oz	430	180	42
(Swanson Hungry Man)	16 1/2 oz	610	315	52
Salmon loaf, 2 x 2 x 3" ✔	1 slice	341	135	40
Salmon				
Atlantic, raw	1 oz	40	15	38
Chinook, smoked	1 oz	33	11	33
Coho/Silver, poached	1 oz	52	19	37
Humpback/Pink, canned	1 oz	39	15	38
Sockeye, broiled	1 oz	62	28	45
Salsa (Taco Bell)	1 serving	18	8	44
Salsa Picante, hot or mild (Del Monte)	1/4 cup	15	0	0
Salt pork, raw	1 oz	212	205	97

FOOD

CALORIES

	AMOUNT	TOTAL	FAT	%FAT
Salt water taffy	1 oz	108	8	7
Saltine crackers, 2" square	2 crackers	25	4	16
Sandwich bread				
white, 4 x 4 x 1/2"	1 slice	60	9	15
whole wheat, 4 x 4 x 1/2"	1 slice	45	9	20
Sandwich spread, with pickle				
regular	1 Tbsp	76	65	86
reduced calorie	1 Tbsp	22	16	73
Sandwich type cookie, chocolate or vanilla	1 cookie	50	19	38
Sangria ✔	1/2 cup	98	0	0
Sapodilla	1 average	140	18	13
Sardines, canned in oil, drained	1 oz	59	29	49
canned in tomato sauce	1 oz	50	31	62
Sauerkraut, canned	1/2 cup	20	tr	tr
Sausage				
(Brown and Serve), browned	1 link	70	54	77
bulk or links, cooked	1 oz	110	81	74
cholesterol free	1 oz	80	45	56
patty (Wendy's)	1 1/2 oz	200	162	81
Polish, 10" x 1 1/4"	8 oz	690	516	75
5 3/8" x 1"	2.7 oz	231	172	74
pork, cooked	1/2 cup	280	211	75
	1 oz	105	79	75
pork, 2 oz (McDonald's)	1 serving	180	147	82
summer, beef stick (Hickory Farms)	1 oz	100	72	72
Scallions, green onions, 3/8" diameter	1 onion	3	tr	tr
Scallopini, veal	1 cup	790	359	45
Scallops				
breaded, fried ✔	1 oz	61	28	46
steamed	1 oz	32	3	9
Scone	1 average	99	54	55
Seafood baskets (Skipper's)				
clam strips and fries	1 basket	1003	630	63
original shrimp and fries	1 basket	723	324	45
Skipper's platter and fries	1 basket	1038	567	55

FOOD
CALORIES

	AMOUNT	TOTAL	FAT	%FAT
Seafood combo basket (Skipper's)				
original shrimp, 1 fish fillet and fries	1 basket	728	333	46
oysters, 1 fish fillet and fries	1 basket	885	396	45
Seltzer water, flavored, sweetened	10 oz	140	0	0
Sesame seeds	1 Tbsp	48	42	88
Seven Grain bread, 4 x 5 1/4 x 3/8"	1 slice	100	9	9
Seven Grain Cereal				
cooked	1 cup	79	10	13
dry	1 cup	504	68	13
Seven layer salad ✔	1/2 cup	181	137	76
Seven Up	12 oz	144	0	0
sugar free	12 oz	4	0	0
Shad, baked	1 oz	57	29	51
Shake 'n Bake mix	1 oz	116	38	33
Shallot bulb, raw, chopped	1 Tbsp	7	tr	tr
Shark, raw	1 oz	37	12	32
Shells, pasta				
cooked	1 cup	100	9	9
dry	1 cup	200	18	9
Sherbet, all varieties	1 cup	270	36	13
Shortbread cookie, 1 5/8" square x 1/4"	1 cookie	37	16	43
Shortcake, plain, 2 1/2" diameter ✔	1 piece	221	108	49
Shortening, vegetable, solid	1 Tbsp	111	111	100
	1 cup	1776	1776	100
Shredded Wheat (Nabisco)				
biscuits	1 biscuit	80	tr	tr
spoon-size	1 cup	136	tr	tr
Shrimp and seafood salad (Skipper's)	1 salad	175	45	26
Shrimp chow mein ✔	1 1/2 cups	455	153	34
Shrimp cocktail ✔	2 oz shrimp	106	9	8
Shrimp crepes (Mrs. Smith's)	2 crepes	305	144	47
Shrimp Foo Yung	1 cup	288	189	66
Shrimp Fried Rice, frozen (Green Giant)	10 oz	300	45	15
Shrimp Newburg ✔	1 salad	572	387	68

FOOD		CALORIES		
	AMOUNT	TOTAL	FAT	%FAT
Shrimp salad				
with mayonnaise	1/2 cup	251	205	82
with Miracle Whip salad dressing	1/2 cup	178	118	66
Shrimp				
breaded, fried, 1 shrimp = 1/2 oz	1 oz	69	31	45
canned	1 oz	28	3	11
steamed, 4 medium = 1 oz	1 oz	28	3	11
Shrimp-avacado salad ✔	1 2/3 cups	295	162	55
Side salad				
(McDonald's)	1 salad	60	30	50
(Hardee's)	1 salad	20	tr	tr
Simple Pleasures, frozen dessert				
chocolate	1 cup	280	tr	tr
strawberry	1 cup	240	tr	tr
Sirloin Enchilada Ranchero, frozen				
(Budget Gourmet Slim Selects)	9 oz	290	135	47
Sirloin Tips dinner, frozen (Healthy Choice)	11 3/4 oz	290	54	19
Sirloin Tips with Burgundy Sauce dinner				
frozen (Budget Gourmet)	11 oz	310	99	32
Skim milk	8 oz	85	tr	tr
Sloppy Joe mixture, without roll	1 cup	568	343	60
Snicker's				
regular size, 2 oz	1 bar	270	125	46
snack size, 1 oz	1 bar	135	58	43
Snickerdoodles ✔	1 cookie	79	27	34
Snow or sugar pea pods, fresh	1/2 cup	26	1	4
Snowball, 2" diameter (Hostess)	1 piece	160	45	28
Soft serve ice cream with cone				
(Dairy Queen)	1 small	140	36	26
	1 regular	240	63	26
	1 large	340	90	26
dipped (Dairy Queen)	1 small	190	80	42
	1 regular	340	144	42
	1 large	510	216	42
(McDonald's)	1 cone	140	41	29

FOOD

CALORIES

	AMOUNT	TOTAL	FAT	%FAT
Soft serve ice cream without cone				
(Dairy Queen)	1 cup	261	78	30
Sole, au Gratin dinner				
frozen (Healthy Choice)	11 1/2 oz	280	45	16
Sole, broiled	1 oz	23	2	9
Sorbet (Dole)	1 cup	240	tr	tr
Sopaipillas, 3" x 3"	1 piece	141	107	76
Sour cream	1 Tbsp	31	27	87
	1 cup	495	432	87
half-and-half	1 Tbsp	21	16	76
	1 cup	335	251	75
Sour cream dressing	1 Tbsp	28	24	86
Sour cream-raisin pie, single crust ✔				
1/6 of 9"	1 piece	683	270	40
1/8 of 9"	1 piece	513	203	40
9", whole	1 pie	4100	1620	40
Sourdough bread	1 slice	76	2	3
Soy milk	1 cup	79	45	57
Soy nuts, snack food	1 cup	63	24	38
Soy sauce, regular or lite	1 Tbsp	10	tr	tr
Soybeans				
sprouted seeds, cooked or raw	1 cup	48	16	33
whole				
cooked	1 cup	234	93	40
dry	1 cup	846	335	40
Spaghetti sauce				
with meat ✔	1 cup	297	167	56
without meat ✔	1 cup	171	72	42
meat flavored (Prego)	1 cup	288	72	25
(Ragú)	1 cup	160	36	23
plain (Ragú)	1 cup	160	54	34
plain or mushroom (Prego)	1 cup	276	72	26
Spaghetti with meatballs ✔	1 cup	332	105	32
frozen (Swanson)	12 1/2 oz	370	144	39
Spaghetti with Meat Sauce				
frozen (Stouffer's)	12 7/8 oz	370	99	27

FOOD		CALORIES		
	AMOUNT	TOTAL	FAT	%FAT
Spaghetti, pasta, cooked				
firm	1 cup	192	6	3
tender	1 cup	155	5	3
Spaghetti, dry	1 lb	1674	49	3
Spaghetti spinach, cooked	1 cup	192	6	3
Spaghetti, whole wheat, cooked				
firm	1 cup	183	13	7
tender	1 cup	152	11	7
Spaghetti, whole wheat, dry	1 lb	1600	117	7
Spam (Hormel)	1 oz	87	67	77
Spanish Rice ✔	1/2 cup	217	81	37
Spareribs, pork, braised	1 oz	113	77	68
Special K (Kellogg's)	1 cup	110	0	0
Special sauce (Wendy's)	1 Tbsp	40	27	68
Spice cake (Betty Crocker)	1 cake	3120	1188	38
1/12	1 piece	260	99	38
Spicy sour hot soup, Chinese	1 cup	79	35	44
Spinach, chopped				
canned, fresh or frozen, cooked	1/2 cup	23	4	17
raw	1 cup	15	tr	tr
Spinach, chopped				
canned, fresh or frozen, cooked	1/2 cup	23	4	17
raw	1 cup	15	tr	tr
Split pea soup				
homemade ✔	1 cup	233	54	23
with water	1 cup	145	27	19
Spongecake				
1/12, without frosting	1 piece	195	37	19
9 3/4" diameter, without frosting	1 cake	2340	444	19
individual size	1 cake	84	14	17
Spoonbread ✔	1/2 cup	234	123	53
Sportsman stick (Hickory Farms)	1 oz	138	90	65
Sprite, regular	12 oz	144	0	0
diet	12 oz	4	0	0
Spritz ✔	1 cookie	81	45	56
Sprouts, alfalfa	1/2 cup	12	1	8

FOOD

CALORIES

	AMOUNT	TOTAL	FAT	%FAT
Squash				
acorn, baked, 1/2 squash	1/2 cup	65	9	14
candied ✔	1/2 squash	164	36	22
summer, all varieties, cooked	1/2 cup	15	tr	tr
winter, all varieties, cooked	1/2 cup	65	4	6
Squid, steamed	1 oz	30	3	10
Starfruit, 4" diameter	1 average	42	3	7
Steak, beef				
cubed, cooked	1 oz	75	40	53
flank, broiled	1 oz	69	38	55
porterhouse, broiled	1 oz	62	28	45
sirloin, broiled	1 oz	58	18	31
T-bone, broiled	1 oz	61	26	43
top loin, broiled	1 oz	57	23	40
top round, broiled	1 oz	54	16	30
Stewed chicken ✔	4 oz meat	167	54	32
Stir'N Streusel cake (Betty Crocker)	1 cake	1440	378	26
1/6, with topping	1 piece	240	63	26
Strawberries				
fresh, large	10 berries	37	5	14
frozen, sliced, sweetened	1/2 cup	140	2	1
whole, sweetened	1/2 cup	112	2	2
Strawberry crepes (Mrs. Smith's)	1 crepe	150	45	30
Strawberry Newtons (Nabisco)	1 cookie	80	18	23
Strawberry Nectar (Kerns)	8 oz	144	0	0
Strawberry pie, single crust ✔				
1/6 of 9"	1 piece	245	88	36
1/8 of 9"	1 piece	184	66	36
9", whole	1 pie	1469	527	36
Strawberry shortcake, with berries, cream ✔	1 piece	380	70	18
Strawberry Shortcake bar, 3 oz (Good Humor)	1 bar	186	108	58
Strawberry topping (Smucker's)	1 Tbsp	40	tr	tr
Strawberry-rhubarb pie ✔				
1/6 of 9"	1 piece	576	228	40
1/8 of 9"	1 piece	432	171	40
9", whole	1 pie	3456	1368	40

FOOD

CALORIES

	AMOUNT	TOTAL	FAT	%FAT
Stroganoff, beef, with noodles ✔	1 1/2 cups	735	495	67
Stuffed cabbage rolls ✔	1 roll	314	180	57
Stuffed cornish game hens ✔	1/2 hen	385	216	56
Stuffed flounder ✔	4 oz fish	311	153	49
Stuffed manicotti ✔	1 each	188	54	29
Stuffed pepper, 2 3/4" long ✔	1 pepper	322	167	52
Stuffed pork chops ✔	1 chop	802	585	73
Stuffing				
cornbread ✔	1/2 cup	257	126	49
dry (Stove Top)	1/2 cup	110	9	8
homemade ✔	1/2 cup	251	138	55
mix, moist, with egg	1/2 cup	198	110	56
Sturgeon				
smoked	1 oz	48	11	23
steamed	1 oz	39	14	36
Submarine roll, 11 1/2 x 3"	1 roll	392	37	9
Sugar cookie, 3" diameter ✔	1 cookie	48	21	44
Sugar				
brown, packed	1 tsp	17	0	0
	1 Tbsp	51	0	0
	1/2 cup	410	0	0
granulated	1 tsp	15	0	0
	1 Tbsp	45	0	0
	1/2 cup	360	0	0
1 packet = 6 grams	1 packet	23	0	0
Sugar, maple, 1 3/4 x 1 1/4 x 1/2"	1 oz	99	0	0
Sugar, powdered, sifted	1/2 cup	193	0	0
Summer sausage, beef stick	1 oz	100	72	72
Sundae, all varieties (Dairy Queen)				
large	1 sundae	440	90	20
regular	1 sundae	310	72	23
small	1 sundae	190	36	19
Sundae, soft serve (McDonald's)				
hot caramel	1 sundae	340	82	24
hot fudge	1 sundae	310	85	27
strawberry	1 sundae	280	66	23

FOOD

CALORIES

	AMOUNT	TOTAL	FAT	%FAT
Sunflower seeds, shelled	1 Tbsp	51	39	76
400 small seeds = 1 oz	1 oz	158	110	70
5.4 oz = 1 cup	1 cup	853	594	70
Sushi over 1/4 cup rice	1 cup	250	6	2
Sweet 'n Sour Chicken with Rice				
frozen (Budget Gourmet)	10 oz	350	63	18
Sweet and Sour Chicken dinner				
frozen (Healthy Choice)	11 1/2 oz	280	18	6
Sweet and sour pork, Chinese	1 cup	344	209	61
Swedish Meatballs with Noodles				
frozen (Budget Gourmet)	10 oz	600	351	59
Sweet potatoes				
boiled or baked, with skin, 5 x 2"	1 potato	170	9	5
candied, 2 x 2 1/2"	1 piece	175	27	15
canned, solid pack	1/2 cup	138	4	3
Sweet roll, commercial, 2 oz	1 roll	178	38	21
Sweet-sour sauce ✔	1/4 cup	99	0	0
Sweetened condensed milk, canned	1 cup	980	243	25
Sweet potato pie, single crust ✔				
1/6 of 9"	1 piece	323	154	48
1/8 of 9"	1 piece	243	116	48
9", whole	1 pie	1938	925	48
Swiss chard, cooked, leaves and stalks	1/2 cup	13	2	15
Swiss cheese	1 oz	105	70	67
Light Naturals (Kraft)	1 oz	90	45	50
reduced fat (Hickory Farm)	1 oz	80	54	68
Swiss cheese food, processed	1 oz	95	63	66
Swiss steak, 3 x 3 x 1/2" ✔	1 piece	214	81	38
dinner, frozen (Swanson)	10 oz	350	99	28
Swordfish, broiled	1 oz	44	13	30
Sylvester Fish Sticks, frozen				
(Tyson Looney Tunes Meals)	7.3 oz	270	99	37
Syrup, chocolate				
fudge type	1 Tbsp	62	23	37
thin type	1 Tbsp	46	4	9

FOOD	AMOUNT	CALORIES		
		TOTAL	FAT	%FAT
Syrup, pancake				
fruit flavored	1 Tbsp	59	0	0
maple flavored	1 Tbsp	59	0	0
reduced sugar, "lite"	1 Tbsp	30	0	

T

FOOD	AMOUNT	TOTAL	FAT	%FAT
Tabasco pepper sauce	1/4 tsp	tr	tr	tr
Tabouli	1/2 cup	112	36	32
Taco (Taco Bell)	1 taco	183	97	53
Bellgrande	1 taco	355	207	58
Light	1 taco	410	259	63
Taco, soft (Taco Bell)	1 taco	228	106	47
supreme	1 taco	275	147	53
Taco				
beef ✔	1 taco	288	153	53
chicken ✔	1 taco	231	90	39
Taco chips, 10 chips = 1 oz (Tostitos)	1 oz	140	72	51
Taco salad ✔	1/2 cup	141	90	64
(Wendy's)	1 salad	660	330	50
Taco salad shell, 2.5 oz	1 shell	421	269	64
Taco salad with shell, with salsa (Taco Bell)	1 salad	941	552	59
without shell, with salsa (Taco Bell)	1 salad	520	283	54
Taco sauce	1/2 cup	28	2	7
hot (Taco Bell)	1 packet	3	tr	tr
regular (Taco Bell)	1 packet	2	tr	tr
Taco shell, hard	1 average	48	20	42
Tahini, sesame seed butter	1 tsp	45	27	60
Tamale pie, without meat ✔	1 cup	176	71	40

FOOD	AMOUNT	CALORIES		
		TOTAL	FAT	%FAT
Tamale ✔				
with beef and sauce	1 tamale	244	98	40
with cheese and sauce	1 tamale	244	93	38
with chicken/sauce, 4" tube	1 tamale	164	65	40
with sauce, without meat, 4" tube	1 tamale	139	57	41
(Old El Paso)	2 tamales	232	114	49
Tangerine, fresh, large	1 tangerine	46	2	4
Tangelo, fresh, medium	1 tangelo	39	1	3
Tangerine juice, canned, unsweetened	8 oz	125	tr	tr
Tapioca, dry	1 cup	535	3	1
	1 Tbsp	30	tr	tr
Tartar sauce, regular	1 Tbsp	75	72	96
Tater Tots, frozen potato (Ore Ida)	4 oz	213	96	45
Tea, brewed	6 oz	2	tr	tr
Tempura ✔	1 cup	264	209	79
Teriyaki Chicken, frozen (Budget Gourmet)	12 oz	360	108	30
Teriyaki sauce	1 Tbsp	17	tr	tr
Tetrazini, chicken	1 cup	442	185	42
Thousand Island salad dressing				
regular	1 Tbsp	80	72	90
reduced calorie	1 Tbsp	25	18	72
(Burger King)	1 packet	240	207	86
(McDonald's)	1 packet	390	338	87
Three bean salad ✔	1/2 cup	153	64	42
Three Musketeers, snack size, 0.8 oz	1 bar	80	18	23
Tilsit cheese	1 oz	97	66	68
Tofu, soybean curd	1/2 cup	81	43	53
	1 lb	331	174	53
2 1/2 x 2 3/4 x 1"	1 piece	86	45	52
Tofutti, frozen dessert				
Lite, Lite	1 cup	180	tr	tr
vanilla, regular	1 cup	400	198	50
Tom Collins	10 oz	180	0	0
Tomatillos	1/2 cup	37	4	11
Tomato aspic salad ✔	1/2 cup	44	1	2

FOOD		CALORIES		
	AMOUNT	TOTAL	FAT	%FAT
Tomato catsup	1 Tbsp	15	tr	tr
	1/2 cup	145	4	3
Tomato juice, canned	8 oz	45	tr	tr
Tomato paste	1 Tbsp	12	tr	tr
	1/2 cup	96	tr	tr
Tomato puree	1/2 cup	49	2	4
	1 Tbsp	6	tr	tr
Tomato sauce, regular or Spanish	1/2 cup	43	3	7
	1 Tbsp	5	tr	tr
Tomato soup				
canned, condensed (Campbell's)	1 cup	180	48	27
with 3.8% milk	1 cup	170	67	39
with skim milk	1 cup	132	18	14
with water	1 cup	90	27	30
cream of, homemade ✔	1 cup	189	99	52
Tomato vegetable noodle soup, with water	1 cup	65	9	14
Tomato vegetable soup, dry, reconstituted	1 cup	56	2	4
Tomatoes				
canned	1/2 cup	25	tr	tr
raw, 3" diameter, whole	1 tomato	25	tr	tr
sliced	3 slices	9	tr	tr
Tonic water (Schweppes)	12 oz	132	0	0
sugar free	12 oz	2	tr	tr
Tootsie Roll, miniature	1 small	24	5	21
Tortellini with Cheese Sauce				
frozen (Budget Gourmet)	5 1/2 oz	180	54	30
Tortellini, Cheese, Alfredo, frozen (Stouffer's)	8 7/8 oz	600	360	60
Tortellini, cooked				
cheese	1 cup	754	108	14
meat	1 cup	754	108	14
Tortilla				
corn, soft, 6" diameter	1 tortilla	63	5	8
flour, soft, 6" diameter	1 tortilla	95	18	19
8" diameter	1 tortilla	127	24	19
taco shell, hard	1 average	48	20	42
whole wheat, soft, 6" diameter	1 tortilla	97	16	16

FOOD	AMOUNT	CALORIES		
		TOTAL	FAT	%FAT
Tossed salad				
with 1 Tbsp dressing	1 cup	112	73	65
without dressing	1 cup	32	3	9
Tostada				
with beef and refried beans	1 tostada	239	130	54
(Taco Bell)	1 tosada	243	100	41
Total (General Mills)	1 cup	110	9	8
Town House crackers (Keebler)	1 cracker	17	9	53
Trail Mix				
regular	1 oz	132	73	55
	1 lb	2112	1168	55
	1/2 cup	330	183	55
Cross Country	1 oz	144	95	66
	1/2 cup	533	351	66
Tropical	1 oz	104	34	33
	1 lb	1644	544	33
	1/2 cup	302	99	33
Triscuit cracker (Nabisco)	1 cracker	21	13	62
Trix (General Mills)	1 cup	110	9	8
Trout, Rainbow, broiled	1 oz	43	11	26
Trout Amandine ✔	4 oz fish	264	180	68
Tuna salad sandwich on white	1 sandwich	320	109	34
Tuna salad, with egg and mayonnaise ✔	1/2 cup	174	97	56
Tuna				
Bluefin, broiled	1 oz	53	16	30
light, canned in oil	1 oz	56	21	38
canned in water	1 oz	37	1	3
white, canned in oil	1 oz	53	21	40
canned in water	1 oz	39	6	15
Tuna-noodle casserole ✔	1 cup	393	168	43
frozen (Swanson)	9 oz	260	99	38
Tuna-stuffed tomatoes ✔	1 salad	263	162	62
Turkey				
breast, barbecued (Louis Rich)	1 oz	40	9	23
dark meat, roasted, without skin	1 oz	58	21	36
diced, dark meat, 1 cup = 4.5 oz	1 cup	261	95	36

FOOD		CALORIES		
	AMOUNT	TOTAL	FAT	%FAT
Turkey (continued)				
diced, white meat, 1 cup = 4.5 oz	1 cup	225	45	20
ground, raw (Golden Farms)	1 oz	40	18	45
ground, 10% fat, cooked	1 oz	51	21	41
15% fat, cooked	1 oz	60	34	57
hickory smoked breast (Louis Rich)	1 oz	35	7	20
honey roasted breast (Louis Rich)	1 oz	35	7	20
light meat, roasted, without skin	1 oz	50	10	20
pressed (Land O'Frost)	1 oz	50	27	54
Turkey bologna	1 oz	57	39	68
Turkey franks, 8 = 1 lb (Louis Rich)	1 frank	130	90	69
Turkey ham	1 oz	37	13	35
Turkey luncheon meat (Land O'Frost)	1 oz	50	27	54
Turkey pastrami (Louis Rich)	1 oz	35	14	40
Turkey roll, light and dark meat	1 oz	42	18	43
Turkey salami (Louis Rich)	1 oz	55	36	65
Turkey sandwich				
club (Hardee's)	1 sandwich	390	144	37
deluxe (Arby's)	1 sandwich	375	149	40
Turkey summer sausage (Louis Rich)	1 oz	55	32	58
Turkey Dijon, frozen (Lean Cuisine)	9 1/2 oz	270	90	33
Turkey Dinner, frozen (Swanson)	9 oz	280	99	35
Turkey Tetrazini, frozen (Stouffer's)	10 oz	380	180	47
Turnip greens, fresh or frozen, cooked	1/2 cup	20	tr	tr
Turnips				
fresh, cooked	1/2 cup	18	tr	tr
raw, diced, 3 1/2 oz = 1 cup	1 cup	40	3	8
Turnover				
apple, 3 oz	1 turnover	255	127	50
cherry, 3 oz	1 turnover	251	127	51
lemon, 3 oz	1 turnover	279	137	49
TVP, textured vegetable protein, dehydrated	1 oz	101	2	2
Twinkie, 3 x 3/4" (Hostess)	1 piece	163	54	33

FOOD

CALORIES

	AMOUNT	TOTAL	FAT	%FAT

V

Vanilla pudding ✔	1/2 cup	271	117	43
Vanilla wafer cookie, 1 3/4" diameter	1 cookie	18	5	28
Veal parmigiana ✔	4 oz meat	408	248	61
dinner, frozen (Swanson)	12 1/4 oz	450	189	42
Veal scallopini ✔	4 oz meat	387	204	53
Veal				
cullets, pan fried	1 oz	58	16	28
loin, boneless, braised	1 oz	64	23	36
shoulder, braised	1 oz	56	16	29
Vegetable beef soup,				
with water (Campbell's)	1 cup	69	9	13
Vegetable juice cocktail	8 oz	40	3	8
Vegetable Omelet mix (Egg Beaters)	1/4 cup	27	0	0
Vegetable stir-fry, meatless ✔	1 cup	94	45	48
Vegetables, frozen				
Japenese style in seasoned sauce	3.3 oz	90	45	50
Oriental style, no sauce	3.3 oz	30	0	0
Vegetarian vegetable soup,				
with water (Campbell's)	1 cup	69	9	13
Venison, cooked	1 oz	57	16	28
raw	1 oz	35	9	26
Vermicelli, coil				
cooked	1 cup	150	9	6
dry	1 cup	200	9	5
Vermouth	1 oz	30	0	0
Vienna bread, 4 3/4 x 4 x 1/2"	1 slice	75	2	3

FOOD

CALORIES

	AMOUNT	TOTAL	FAT	%FAT
Vinaigrette dressing ✔	1 Tbsp	82	81	99
Lite (McDonald's)	1 packet	60	18	30
Vinegar				
cider or white distilled	1 Tbsp	tr	tr	tr
rice, regular (Marukan)	1 Tbsp	1	0	0
rice, seasoned (Marukan)	1 Tbsp	30	0	0
Vitari, frozen fruit treat	1 cup	160	0	0
Vodka, 86 proof	1 oz	74	0	0

W

	AMOUNT	TOTAL	FAT	%FAT
Waffle				
4" diameter (Eggo)	1 waffle	120	45	38
homemade, 5 1/2" diameter ✔	1 waffle	209	67	32
Waldorf salad ✔	1/2 cup	79	56	71
Walnuts, black, halves				
14 = 1 oz	1 oz	179	156	87
4.4 oz = 1 cup	1 cup	788	668	85
English, halves, 14 = 1 oz	1 oz	185	164	89
3.5 oz = 1 cup	1 cup	648	574	89
Wasa Crisp bread				
Hearty Rye	1 cracker	45	tr	tr
Lite Rye	1 cracker	25	tr	tr
Sesame Wheat	1 cracker	50	18	36
Water chestnuts, Chinese, raw	4 nuts	20	1	5
Watercress, raw	10 sprigs	2	tr	tr
Watermelon, fresh				
4 x 8" wedge	1 wedge	110	1	1
diced	1/2 cup	21	1	5

FOOD | CALORIES

	AMOUNT	TOTAL	FAT	%FAT
Welsh Rarebit ✔	1/4 cup	295	162	55
Whaler fish sandwich (Burger King)	1 sandwich	488	243	50
Wheat berries, cooked	1 cup	221	16	7
dry	1 cup	578	42	7
Wheat bran, unprocessed or miller's	1 cup	121	23	19
	1 Tbsp	8	tr	tr
Wheat Chex (Ralston)	1 cup	150	0	0
Wheat germ	1 Tbsp	23	6	26
2 oz = 1 cup	1 cup	368	101	27
Wheat Thin cracker (Nabisco)	1 cracker	9	3	33
Cheese	1 cracker	8	3	38
Nutty	1 cracker	11	6	55
Wheat, cracked, cooked	1 cup	227	8	4
dry	1 cup	509	30	6
Wheat, rolled, cooked	1 cup	180	8	4
dry	1 cup	405	18	4
Wheat, whole grain, cooked	1 cup	243	8	3
Wheatena, cooked	1 cup	150	4	3
dry	1 cup	600	20	3
Wheaties (General Mills)	1 cup	104	1	1
Wheatsworth cracker (Nabisco)	1 cracker	14	6	43
Whiskey, 86 proof	1 oz	74	0	0
White bread				
4 1/2 x 4 x 1/2"	1 slice	70	9	13
crumbs	1 cup	120	9	8
cubes	1 cup	80	9	11
White cake (Betty Crocker)	1 cake	2760	972	35
1/12, without frosting	1 piece	230	81	35
1/12, with 3 Tbsp chocolate frosting	1 piece	410	132	32
White sauce, medium ✔	1 Tbsp	27	18	67
	1/4 cup	107	73	68
White wine punch ✔	4 oz	91	0	0
Whitefish, smoked	1 oz	31	2	6
Whiting, broiled	1 oz	33	4	12
Whole wheat bread, 4 1/2 x 4 x 1/2"	1 slice	60	9	15
100% stone ground, 5 x 4 1/2 x 1/2"	1 slice	100	9	9

FOOD

CALORIES

	AMOUNT	TOTAL	FAT	%FAT
Whole wheat noodles, homemade ✔	1/2 cup	88	9	10
Whole wheat roll	1 average	90	9	10
Whopper (Burger King)	1 burger	628	324	52
with cheese	1 burger	711	387	54
Wild rice, cooked	1 cup	141	3	2
dry	1 cup	396	7	2
Wine cooler	12 oz	184	0	0
Wine				
dessert, 18% alcohol	4 oz	160	0	0
port, 15% alcohol	4 oz	180	0	0
red and white table, 12% alcohol	4 oz	116	0	0
sherry	4 oz	168	0	0
Winter squash, cooked	1/2 cup	65	4	6
Won Ton soup ✔	1 cup	205	31	15
Won Ton, pork, fried	1 piece	59	40	68
Worcestershire sauce	1 tsp	4	0	0

Y

	AMOUNT	TOTAL	FAT	%FAT
Yams, boiled or baked, with skin	1/2 cup	105	2	2
Yeast, baker's				
compressed	1 cake	10	tr	tr
dry	1 Tbsp	23	tr	tr
Yeast, brewer's, dry	1 Tbsp	25	tr	tr
Yellow cake (Betty Crocker)				
1/12, without frosting	1 piece	150	33	22
without frosting	1 cake	1800	396	22
Yogurt almonds	1 oz	150	90	60

FOOD	AMOUNT	CALORIES		
		TOTAL	FAT	%FAT
Yogurt (Yoplait)				
breakfast style	6 oz	220	27	12
custard style	6 oz	190	36	19
fruit flavors, light	6 oz	90	5	6
plain	6 oz	120	27	23
Yogurt, low-fat				
fruit flavored	1 cup	240	27	11
plain	1 Tbsp	9	2	22
	1 cup	140	31	22
vanilla, lemon, or coffee	1 cup	200	27	14
Yogurt, non-fat				
plain	1 cup	110	tr	tr
with fruit	1 cup	150	tr	tr
Yogurt, whole milk	1 cup	150	63	42
Yogurt, frozen, low-fat				
(Dannon)	1 cup	240	26	11
(Honey Hill Farms)	1 cup	210	56	27
(I Can't Believe It's Yogurt)	1 cup	288	65	23
(TCBY)	1 cup	240	72	30
(Tuscan Farms)	1 cup	220	18	8
Gourmet (Yo Cream)	1 cup	240	72	30
Yogurt, frozen, non-fat				
(I Can't Believe It's Yogurt	1 cup	224	18	8
(TCBY)	1 cup	200	18	9
Lite (Yo Cream)	1 cup	200	34	17
Yogurt, frozen, non-fat, sugar free				
(Honey Hilll Farms)	1 cup	80	tr	tr

FOOD

CALORIES

	AMOUNT	TOTAL	FAT	%FAT

Z

	AMOUNT	TOTAL	FAT	%FAT
Zucchini bread ✔				
5 x 4 x 1/2"	1/18 loaf	153	59	39
9 x 5 x 4 1/2"	1 loaf	2771	1078	39
Zucchini Lasagna, frozen (Lean Cuisine)	11 oz	260	63	24
Zucchini squash				
cooked, diced	1/2 cup	13	tr	tr
raw, sliced or diced	1/2 cup	11	tr	tr

FOOD		CALORIES		
	AMOUNT	TOTAL	FAT	%FAT

FOOD		CALORIES		
	AMOUNT	TOTAL	FAT	%FAT

FOOD		CALORIES		
	AMOUNT	TOTAL	FAT	%FAT

FOOD		CALORIES		
	AMOUNT	TOTAL	FAT	%FAT

FOOD GROUP LIST

FOOD		CALORIES		
	AMOUNT	TOTAL	FAT	%FAT

BEVERAGES, ALCOHOLIC

FOOD	AMOUNT	TOTAL	FAT	%FAT
Ale	12 oz	147	0	0
Baileys Irish Cream	1 oz	118	25	21
Beer, light				
Bud Light (Budweiser)	12 oz	108	0	0
Lite (Miller)	12 oz	96	0	0
Oly Gold (Olympia)	12 oz	70	0	0
Beer, regular	12 oz	168	0	0
Bloody Mary	6 oz	160	0	0
Brandy	1 oz	73	0	0
Brandy Alexander, with 3 Tbsp cream	3 oz	237	100	42
Champagne	4 oz	84	0	0
Creme DeMenthe	1 oz	101	0	0
Curacao, orange flavored liqueur	1 oz	81	0	0
Daiquiri	3 oz	122	0	0
Eggnog (4 oz) with 1 oz rum	5 oz	245	85	35
Gin, 86 proof	1 oz	70	0	0
Grasshopper cocktail with cream	3 oz	264	158	60
Hot buttered rum mix ✔	1/3 cup	360	162	45
Irish coffee ✔	6 oz	154	81	53
Kahlua, 63 proof	1 oz	107	0	0
Manhattan cocktail	4 oz	186	0	0
Martini cocktail	4 oz	160	0	0
Old Fashioned cocktail	6 oz	269	0	0
Rum, 86 proof	1 oz	74	0	0
Sangria ✔	1/2 cup	98	0	0

Abbreviations and symbols:

lb = pound	oz = ounce	Tbsp = Tablespoon
tsp = teaspoon	tr = trace	pkg = package

✔ = homemade, a standard cookbook recipe we have not changed to lower fat. Use the check to remind yourself *you can modify recipes.* See page 16 for tips on lowering fat in any recipe without losing quality or flavor.

FOOD

CALORIES

	AMOUNT	TOTAL	FAT	%FAT
Tom Collins	10 oz	180	0	0
Vermouth	1 oz	30	0	0
Vodka, 86 proof	1 oz	74	0	0
Whiskey, 86 proof	1 oz	74	0	0
White wine punch ✔	4 oz	91	0	0
Wine cooler	12 oz	184	0	0
Wine				
dessert, 18% alcohol	4 oz	160	0	0
Port, 15% alcohol	4 oz	180	0	0
red and white table, 12% alcohol	4 oz	116	0	0
Sherry	4 oz	168	0	0

BEVERAGES, NONALCOHOLIC

	AMOUNT	TOTAL	FAT	%FAT
Cider, apple	8 oz	123	0	0
Club Soda (Schweppes)	12 oz	tr	0	0
Coca Cola	12 oz	144	0	0
Cocoa				
baking	1 Tbsp	21	15	71
instant				
reconstituted with water (Swiss Miss)	8 oz	146	36	25
sugar free, reconstituted (Alba)	8 oz	60	0	0
sugar free, reconstituted (Swiss Miss)	8 oz	64	0	0
with marshmallow, reconstituted				
with water	8 oz	146	36	25
with powdered skim milk	4 tsp	109	9	8
Coffee, instant granules	1 tsp	4	0	0
Coffee, regular or decaffeinated	6 oz	4	tr	tr
Cola type beverages	12 oz	145	0	0
Eggnog (nonalcoholic)	8 oz	340	171	50

FOOD

CALORIES

	AMOUNT	TOTAL	FAT	%FAT
Fruit punch (Hawaiian Punch)	8 oz	120	0	0
"lite" (Hawaiian Punch)	8 oz	107	0	0
Fruit-flavored carbonated sodas	12 oz	166	0	0
sugar free	12 oz	3	0	0
Ginger ale (Schweppes)	12 oz	132	0	0
sugar free	12 oz	4	0	0
Hot mulled cider ✔	1 cup	176	0	0
International coffees	6 oz	55	24	44
sugar free, all varieties	6 oz	30	18	60
Kool aid, diluted				
sugar free	8 oz	2	0	0
with sugar	8 oz	90	0	0
Mineral water	8 oz	0	0	0
Mineral water and juice soda	10 oz	124	0	0
Orange drink (Hi-C)	8 oz	136	0	0
Pepsi Cola	12 oz	156	0	0
Pepsi Light	12 oz	1	0	0
Postum, instant, powder	2 Tbsp	36	tr	tr
Root beer	12 oz	150	0	0
sugar free	12 oz	1	0	0
Seltzer water, flavored, sweetened	10 oz	140	0	0
Seven Up	12 oz	144	0	0
sugar free	12 oz	4	0	0
Sprite, regular	12 oz	144	0	0
diet	12 oz	4	0	0
Strawberry Nectar (Kerns)	8 oz	144	0	0
Tea, brewed	6 oz	2	tr	tr
Tonic water (Schweppes)	12 oz	132	0	0
sugar free	12 oz	2	tr	tr

FOOD		CALORIES		
	AMOUNT	TOTAL	FAT	%FAT

BREADS

Apple-raisin muffins ✔	1 muffin	201	81	40
Bagel with egg, 3 1/2" diameter, plain	1 bagel	180	13	7
Bagel without egg, 3 1/2" diameter				
garlic	1 bagel	180	9	5
onion	1 bagel	180	9	5
plain	1 bagel	170	9	5
raisin honey	1 bagel	180	9	5
Banana bread				
5 x 4 1/2 x 1/2"	1/18 loaf	136	52	38
9 x 5 x 4 1/2" loaf	1 loaf	2441	941	39
Banana nut bread ✔	1/16 loaf	154	54	35
Biscuits				
buttermilk	1 biscuit	82	37	45
2" diameter	1 biscuit	105	45	43
refrigerator (Pillsbury)	1 biscuit	100	36	36
Blueberry pancake, 4" diameter	1 pancake	134	27	20
Boston brown bread, canned				
3 1/4 x 1/2"	1 slice	95	8	8
Branola bread, 5 x 3 1/2 x 1/2"	1 slice	100	9	9
Bread crumbs				
dry, grated	1 cup	346	36	10
white, fresh	1 cup	120	9	8
Bread				
rye, 4 3/4 x 3 3/4 x 7/16"	1 slice	60	tr	tr
white, 4 1/2 x 4 x 1/2"	1 slice	70	9	13
white, sandwich, 4 x 4 x 1/2"	1 slice	60	9	15
whole wheat, 4 1/2 x 4 x 1/2"	1 slice	60	9	15
whole wheat, sandwich, 4 x 4 x 1/2"	1 slice	45	9	20
whole wheat, 100% stone gound				
5 x 4 1/2 x 1/2"	1 slice	100	9	9
Bread, Light (Wonder)				
Oatmeal, 4 x 4 x 1/2"	1 slice	40	4	10
Sourdough, 4 x 4 x 3/4"	1 slice	40	4	10
Wheat, 3 1/2 x 4 x 1/2	1 slice	40	4	10

FOOD		CALORIES		
	AMOUNT	TOTAL	FAT	%FAT
Bread, toasted				
white, 4 1/2 x 4 x 1/2"	1 slice	70	9	13
whole wheat, 4 1/2 x 4 x 1/2	1 slice	60	9	15
Buckwheat pancakes				
4" diameter	1 pancake	108	46	43
6" diameter	1 pancake	146	59	40
Bun, hamburger or frankfurter	1 bun	110	18	16
Buttermilk biscuit	1 average	82	37	45
Buttermilk oat bran bread, 4 x 5 x 1/2"	1 slice	80	18	23
Buttermilk pancake				
4" diameter	1 pancake	110	28	25
5" diameter (Krusteaz)	1 pancake	103	15	15
Buttermilk waffle mix, dry				
(Aunt Jemima)	1 cup	510	27	5
Buttermilk waffles, frozen	1 medium	90	24	27
Cardamom bread ✔	1 piece	89	27	30
Cheese bread ✔	1/16 loaf	70	18	26
Cinnamon roll, plain, small				
3" diameter (Pillsbury)	1 roll	145	56	39
homemade ✔	1 roll	176	45	26
Coffeecake				
2 3/4" square	1 piece	230	62	27
8 x 5 1/2 x 1 1/4"	1 cake	1385	361	26
Cornbread				
3" square ✔	1 piece	193	60	31
from mix, 1/12 pkg (General Mills)	1 piece	160	45	28
Cracked wheat bread, 4 1/2 x 4 1/2"	1 slice	65	8	12
Crepes, strawberry (Mrs. Smith's)	1 crepe	150	45	30
without filling, 6" diameter	1 crepe	58	24	41
Croissant, frozen				
1 oz (Sara Lee)	1 small	109	55	50
1.5 oz (Sara Lee)	1 medium	170	81	48
Croissant, homemade ✔	1 small	100	54	54
Croutons	1 Tbsp	37	2	5
Crumpet, 3" diameter	1 roll	129	27	21
Dinner rolls ✔	1 roll	98	27	28

FOOD

CALORIES

	AMOUNT	TOTAL	FAT	%FAT
Dumpling, 2" diameter ✔	1 dumpling	48	29	60
Egg bread ✔	1 slice	119	18	15
English muffin	1 muffin	160	9	6
cinnamon raisin	1 muffin	170	9	5
oat nut bran	1 muffin	160	18	11
sourdough	1 muffin	140	9	6
Frankfurter bun, 5 x 1 3/4"	1 bun	110	18	16
French bread, 5 x 2 1/2 x 1"	1 slice	100	8	8
French toast				
4 1/2 x 4 1/2" ✔	1 slice	119	30	25
4 x 4" (Aunt Jemima)	1 slice	56	15	27
frozen (Eggo)	1 slice	72	17	24
Frozen bread dough, honey wheat (Rhodes)	1/14 loaf	75	5	7
	1 loaf	1050	63	6
Frozen bread dough, white (Rhodes)	1/14 loaf	80	5	7
	1 loaf	1120	63	6
Frozen dinner roll, white (Rhodes)	1 roll	85	27	32
Garlic bread ✔	2 slices	145	81	56
German Stollen ✔	1 slice	94	27	29
Hamburger bun, 4" diameter				
plain	1 bun	110	18	16
sesame seed	1 bun	150	18	12
Hoagie roll, 11 1/2 x 3"	1 roll	392	37	9
Honey Wheat Berry Bread, 3 3/4 x 3 3/4 x 1/2"	1 slice	90	9	10
Hot cross buns	1 average	111	29	26
Hush puppies, deep fried, 1 1/2" diameter	1 piece	51	16	31
Italian bread, 4 1/2 x 3 1/2 x 1"	1 slice	85	tr	tr
Kuchen ✔	1 piece	225	63	28
Lefse, 10" diameter	1 lefse	79	15	19
Less Bread	1 slice	40	tr	tr
Measure Up Bread	1 slice	40	18	45
Muffin, bran, from mix (Duncan Hines)	1 muffin	100	27	27
Muffins, 3" diameter				
blueberry	1 muffin	298	172	58
bran with raisins	1 muffin	271	58	21

FOOD

CALORIES

	AMOUNT	TOTAL	FAT	%FAT
Muffins, 3" diameter (continued)				
corn	1 muffin	215	92	43
oat bran	1 muffin	290	86	30
pumpkin with raisins	1 muffin	287	97	34
Muffins, 4" diameter				
blueberry	1 muffin	397	229	58
bran with raisins	1 muffin	361	77	21
corn	1 muffin	287	122	43
oat bran	1 muffin	387	115	30
pumpkin with raisins	1 muffin	382	130	34
Oat bran bread, 4 1/4 x 5 x 3/4"	1 slice	84	9	11
Oat nut bread, 4 x 5 x 1/2"	1 slice	100	18	18
Pancake				
4" diameter ✔	1 pancake	104	29	28
from "complete" mix, 4" diameter	1 pancake	70	27	39
from mix				
4" diameter	1 pancake	122	36	30
6" diameter	1 pancake	164	48	29
blueberrry, 4" diameter	1 pancake	134	27	20
buckwheat, 4" diameter	1 pancake	108	46	43
buckwheat, 6" diameter	1 pancake	146	59	40
Pita/pocket bread, white or whole wheat	1 bread	163	7	4
Popover ✔	1 average	112	41	37
Potato bread ✔	1 slice	92	9	10
Potato pancakes, 8" diameter ✔	1 pancake	495	113	23
Poulsbo bread, 4 1/2 x 4 x 1/2"	1 slice	105	14	13
Pretzels, soft	1 pretzel	158	27	17
Pumpernickel bread, 5 x 4 x 3/8"	1 slice	80	tr	tr
Pumpkin bread				
5 x 4 1/2 x 1/2" ✔	1/18 loaf	168	56	33
9 x 5 x 4 1/2" ✔	1 loaf	3032	1014	33
Raisin bread, 4 x 3 1/2 x 1/2"	1 slice	65	8	12
Roll, hard, 3 3/4" diameter	1 roll	156	9	6
Roll, onion, 4" diameter	1 roll	190	18	9

FOOD   CALORIES

	AMOUNT	TOTAL	FAT	%FAT
Roll, soft				
2" square or cloverleaf	1 roll	83	14	17
whole wheat	1 average	90	9	10
dinner ✔	1 roll	98	27	28
Rye bread, 4 3/4 x 3 3/4 x 7/16"	1 slice	60	tr	tr
Sandwich bread				
white, 4 x 4 x 1/2"	1 slice	60	9	15
whole wheat, 4 x 4 x 1/2"	1 slice	45	9	20
Scone	1 average	99	54	55
Seven Grain bread, 4 x 5 1/4 x 3/8"	1 slice	100	9	9
Sourdough bread	1 slice	76	2	3
Spoonbread ✔	1/2 cup	234	123	53
Strawberry crepes (Mrs. Smith's)	1 crepe	150	45	30
Stuffing				
cornbread ✔	1/2 cup	257	126	49
dry (Stove Top)	1/2 cup	110	9	8
homemade ✔	1/2 cup	251	138	55
mix, moist, with egg	1/2 cup	198	110	56
Submarine roll, 11 1/2 x 3"	1 roll	392	37	9
Tortilla				
corn, soft, 6" diameter	1 tortilla	63	5	8
flour, soft, 6" diameter	1 tortilla	95	18	19
flour, soft, 8" diameter	1 tortilla	127	24	19
taco shell, hard	1 average	48	20	42
whole wheat, soft, 6" diameter	1 tortilla	97	16	16
Vienna bread, 4 3/4 x 4 x 1/2"	1 slice	75	2	3
Waffle				
4" diameter (Eggo)	1 waffle	120	45	38
homemade, 5 1/2" diameter ✔	1 waffle	209	67	32
White bread				
4 1/2 x 4 x 1/2"	1 slice	70	9	13
crumbs	1 cup	120	9	8
cubes	1 cup	80	9	11
Whole wheat bread				
4 1/2 x 4 x 1/2"	1 slice	60	9	15
100% stone ground, 5 x 4 1/2 x 1/2"	1 slice	100	9	9

FOOD

CALORIES

	AMOUNT	TOTAL	FAT	%FAT
Whole wheat roll	1 average	90	9	10
Yeast, baker's				
compressed	1 cake	10	tr	tr
dry	1 Tbsp	23	tr	tr
Yeast, brewer's, dry	1 Tbsp	25	tr	tr
Zucchini bread ✔				
5 x 4 x 1/2"	1/18 loaf	153	59	39
9 x 5 x 4 1/2"	1 loaf	2771	1078	39

CAKE FROSTINGS

	AMOUNT	TOTAL	FAT	%FAT
Butter with powdered sugar ✔	1 Tbsp	60	17	28
	1 cup	944	272	29
Chocolate and vanilla, Ready to Spread	1 Tbsp	60	24	40
	16 oz	1920	756	39
Chocolate fudge ✔	1 Tbsp	62	22	35
Cream cheese with nuts, mix (Betty Crocker)	1 Tbsp	75	27	36
	1 pkg	1800	648	36
Cream cheese				
homemade ✔	1 Tbsp	63	20	32
Ready to Spread	1 Tbsp	64	24	38
	16 oz	2040	756	37
German chocolate ✔	1 Tbsp	70	50	71
Seven minute ✔	1 Tbsp	45	0	0

FOOD

CALORIES

	AMOUNT	TOTAL	FAT	%FAT

CAKES

	AMOUNT	TOTAL	FAT	%FAT
Angel food cake				
mix, 1/12 of 9 3/4"	1 piece	135	tr	tr
9 3/4" diameter tube	1 cake	1620	1	tr
Applesauce coffee cake ✔	1/8 cake	307	144	47
Applesauce spice cake, 3 x 3 x 1" ✔	1 piece	136	90	66
Black Forest cake,				
1/12, with frosting ✔	1 piece	661	31	5
Carrot cake, 1/12, without frosting				
(Betty Crocker)	1 piece	260	108	42
Carrot cake, with cream cheese frosting,				
2" square	1 piece	334	157	47
without frosting (Betty Crocker)	1 cake	3120	1296	42
Cheesecake				
1/8 of 8" diameter ✔	1 piece	414	251	61
8" diameter ✔	1 cake	3312	2008	61
with cherry sauce ✔	1/12 cake	482	261	54
Classic, snack size (Sara Lee)	1 cake	200	126	63
Chiffon cake, 1/12 of 10" tube ✔	1 piece	287	109	38
Chocolate fudge cake				
without frosting (Betty Crocker)	1 cake	3000	1188	40
1/12, with 3 Tbsp frosting	1 piece	436	165	38
1/12, without frosting (Betty Crocker)	1 piece	250	99	40
Chocolate, bitter or baking	1 oz	142	135	95
Chocolate, Lights, snack size (Hostess)	1.25 oz	110	9	8
Cocoa, baking	1 Tbsp	21	15	71
Coffeecake				
2 3/4" square	1 piece	230	62	27
8 x 5 1/2 x 1 1/4"	1 cake	1385	361	26
Cupcake, plain, from mix, 2 1/2" diameter	1 cupcake	88	27	31
Devil's Food cake				
without frosting (Betty Crocker)	1 cake	3120	1296	42
1/12, with 3 Tbsp 7 minute frosting	1 piece	395	108	27
1/12, without frosting (Betty Crocker)	1 piece	260	108	42
cupcake, 2 1/2" diameter, plain	1 cupcake	120	34	28

FOOD

CALORIES

	AMOUNT	TOTAL	FAT	%FAT
Fruitcake ✔				
dark, 7" diameter	1 cake	5216	1888	36
dark, 1/16 of 7" diameter	1 piece	326	118	36
light	1/36 cake	234	72	31
Fudge Cakes, snack size (Sara Lee)	1 cake	190	90	47
German chocolate cake				
1/12, without frosting (Betty Crocker)	1 piece	260	99	38
1/12, with 3 Tbsp frosting	1 piece	470	249	53
without frosting (Betty Crocker)	1 cake	3120	1188	38
Gingerbread, plain				
1/9 of 8" square	1 piece	175	34	19
8" square	1 cake	1575	306	19
Golden cake (Betty Crocker)				
1/12, without frosting	1 piece	200	72	36
whole, without frosting	1 cake	2400	864	36
Jelly roll ✔	1/10 cake	161	27	17
Pineapple upside down cake,				
1/9 of 8" square	1 piece	270	90	33
8" square	1 cake	2430	810	33
Pound cake				
1/12 of loaf	1 slice	160	84	53
8 1/2 x 3 1/2 x 3 1/4"	1 loaf	1920	1008	53
snack size (Sara Lee)	1 cake	200	99	50
Shortcake, plain, 2 1/2" diameter ✔	1 piece	221	108	49
Spice cake (Betty Crocker)	1 cake	3120	1188	38
1/12	1 piece	260	99	38
Spongecake				
1/12, without frosting	1 piece	195	37	19
9 3/4" diameter, without frosting	1 cake	2340	444	19
individual size	1 cake	84	14	17
Stir 'N Streusel cake (Betty Crocker)	1 cake	1440	378	26
1/6, with topping	1 piece	240	63	26
Strawberry shortcake, with berries, cream ✔	1 piece	380	70	18
White cake (Betty Crocker)	1 cake	2760	972	35
1/12, without frosting	1 piece	230	81	35
1/12, with 3 Tbsp chocolate frosting	1 piece	410	132	32

FOOD

CALORIES

	AMOUNT	TOTAL	FAT	%FAT
Yellow cake (Betty Crocker)				
1/12, without frosting	1 piece	150	33	22
without frosting	1 cake	1800	396	22

CANDIES

	AMOUNT	TOTAL	FAT	%FAT
Almond bark, white dipping chocolate	1 oz	82	14	17
Almond Joy, 1.76 oz	1 bar	250	126	50
Almond Roca	1 oz	164	99	60
Butterscotch candy, hard	1 piece	20	2	10
Butterscotch chips, 3 oz = 1/2 cup	1/2 cup	456	237	52
60 pieces = 1 oz	1 oz	152	79	52
Candied fruit				
cherry, for baking	1 cherry	12	tr	tr
citron, for fruit cake	1 oz	89	1	1
pineapple slice	1 slice	120	2	2
Candy, hard, 1/4 oz	1 piece	25	0	0
sugar free	1 piece	25	0	0
Caramels, plain or chocolate (Kraft)	1 piece	35	9	26
Carmel apples ✔	1 apple	427	90	21
Carmel corn ✔	1 cup	199	81	41
Carob covered almonds	1 oz	150	108	72
Carob drops/stars	1 oz	116	14	12
Chocolate bar				
large size, 8 oz (Hershey)	1 bar	1200	648	54
regular size, 1.5 oz (Hershey)	1 bar	220	117	53
with almonds	1 bar	230	126	55
Chocolate chips, 1 pkg	12 oz	1720	1024	60
3 oz = 1/2 cup	1/2 cup	430	256	60
Chocolate coated creams, 1 piece = 1/2 oz	1 piece	57	20	35
Chocolate coated nougat with carmel	1 oz	118	35	30
Chocolate coated peanuts	1 oz	160	101	63

FOOD

CALORIES

	AMOUNT	TOTAL	FAT	%FAT
Chocolate covered cherries	1 oz	126	36	29
Chocolate covered coconut, candy	1 oz	124	45	36
Chocolate, bitter or baking	1 oz	142	135	95
Corn candy	1/2 cup	364	18	5
Fudge, chocolate, with walnuts, 1" cube	1 piece	89	33	37
Fruit Gems (Sunkist)	1 wafer	31	tr	tr
Gum drops	1 piece	7	tr	tr
	1 oz	98	3	3
Jelly beans, 10 pieces = 1 oz	1 oz	101	1	1
2 oz = 1/4 cup	1/4 cup	202	3	1
Kisses (Hershey)	1 kiss	25	14	56
6 kisses = 1 oz	1 oz	150	84	56
Licorice, stick, 0.35 oz	1 average	35	tr	tr
Life Saver	1 average	8	tr	tr
M & M's Peanut Candies	1 oz	143	64	45
	1 lb	2288	1024	45
M & M's Plain Candies	1 oz	142	53	37
	1 lb	2240	864	39
Maltballs, carob-coated	1 oz	108	19	18
Marshmallows, 1 x 1 x 1"	1 piece	18	tr	tr
Milky Way, regular size, 2 oz	1 bar	260	81	31
snack size, 0.8 oz	1 bar	100	36	36
Mounds, 1.90 oz	1 bar	260	126	48
Peanut brittle	1 oz	120	27	23
Peanut Butter Cup (Reese's)	1 average	86	47	55
Peanuts, carob coated	1 oz	140	73	52
yogurt coated	1 oz	129	78	60
Peppermint patty, chocolate covered	1 oz	116	27	23
Raisins, chocolate coated	1 oz	120	36	30
yogurt coated	1 oz	120	36	30
Reese's Pieces	1 oz	141	51	36
Rolo caramels	1 oz	140	56	40
Salt water taffy	1 oz	108	8	7
Snicker's, regular size, 2 oz	1 bar	270	125	46
snack size, 1 oz	1 bar	135	58	43
Three Musketeers, snack size, 0.8 oz	1 bar	80	18	23

FOOD

CALORIES

	AMOUNT	TOTAL	FAT	%FAT
Tootsie Roll, miniature	1 small	24	5	21
Yogurt almonds	1 oz	150	90	60

CEREALS, COOKED

	AMOUNT	TOTAL	FAT	%FAT
Cornmeal, yellow or white				
cooked	1 cup	120	5	4
dry	1 cup	530	16	3
Cream of Rice, cooked	1 cup	160	tr	tr
Cream of Wheat, cooked	1 cup	133	4	3
Farina, quick cook or regular, cooked	1 cup	105	2	2
Grits, cooked	1 cup	125	tr	tr
Millet, cooked	1 cup	165	13	8
dry	1 cup	660	53	8
Oatmeal, quick or old fashioned				
cooked	1 cup	148	25	17
dry	1 cup	333	57	17
Oatmeal, instant, cooked, 1 packet				
apples and cinnamon	3/4 cup	120	9	8
maple and brown sugar	3/4 cup	150	18	12
raisin, date and walnut	3/4 cup	140	36	26
regular	3/4 cup	90	18	20
Rolled wheat, cooked	1 cup	180	8	4
dry	1 cup	405	18	4
Seven Grain Cereal, cooked	1 cup	79	10	13
dry	1 cup	504	68	13
Wheatena, cooked	1 cup	150	4	3
dry	1 cup	600	20	3

FOOD   CALORIES

	AMOUNT	TOTAL	FAT	%FAT

CEREALS, READY-TO-EAT

	AMOUNT	TOTAL	FAT	%FAT
All Bran (Kellogg's)	1 cup	210	27	13
Almond Delight (Ralston)	1 cup	147	11	7
Apple Jacks (Kellogg's)	1 cup	110	0	0
Bran Buds (Kellogg's)	1 cup	210	27	13
Bran cereal with raisins	1 cup	145	9	6
Bran Checks (Ralston)	1 cup	165	12	7
Bran Flakes, 40%	1 cup	105	9	9
Cheerios, regular or Apple Cinnamon (General Mills)	1 cup	88	14	16
Corn Chex (Ralston)	1 cup	110	0	0
Corn Flakes (Kellogg's)	1 cup	100	0	0
Cracklin' Oat Bran (Kellogg's)	1 cup	220	72	33
Crispix (Kellogg's)	1 cup	110	0	0
Crispy Wheat and Raisins (General Mills)	1 cup	145	12	8
Frosted Mini Wheats (Kellogg's)	1 cup	200	0	0
Fruit and Fiber, all varieties (Post)	1 cup	180	18	10
Fruit Loops (Kellogg's)	1 cup	110	9	8
Fruit Muesli (Ralston)	1 cup	300	54	18
Golden Grahams (General Mills)	1 cup	146	12	8
Granola				
100% Natural (Quaker Oats)	1 cup	560	212	38
coconut-cashew	1 cup	560	216	39
honey	1 cup	440	144	33
plain (Nature Valley)	1 cup	390	189	48
with cinnamon, raisins (Nature Valley)	1 cup	512	176	34
Grape Nuts, 1 cup = 4 oz (Post)	1 cup	440	tr	tr
Honey Nut Cherrios (General Mills)	1 cup	147	9	6
Just Right (Kellogg's)	1 cup	150	0	0
Kix (General Mills)	1 cup	73	6	8
Mueslix , Bran (Kellogg's)	1 cup	280	36	13
Nutri-Grain Almond Raisin (Kellogg's)	1 cup	186	24	13
Nutri-Grain Wheat (Kellogg's)	1 cup	165	0	0

FOOD		CALORIES		
	AMOUNT	TOTAL	FAT	%FAT
Oat Bran Flakes (Kellogg's)	1 cup	200	14	7
Oat Bran Options (Ralston)	1 cup	130	9	7
Post Toasties (Post)	1 cup	80	tr	tr
Product 19 (Kellogg's)	1 cup	100	0	0
Puffed Rice (Quaker)	1 cup	51	1	2
Puffed Wheat (Quaker)	1 cup	53	2	4
Raisin Bran (Kellogg's)	1 cup	150	11	7
Raisin Squares (Kellogg's)	1 cup	180	0	0
Rice Chex (Ralston)	1 cup	96	0	0
Rice Krispies (Kellogg's)	1 cup	110	0	0
Shredded Wheat, biscuits (Nabisco)	1 biscuit	80	tr	tr
spoon-size (Nabisco)	1 cup	136	tr	tr
Special K (Kellogg's)	1 cup	110	0	0
Total (General Mills)	1 cup	110	9	8
Trix (General Mills)	1 cup	110	9	8
Wheat Chex (Ralston)	1 cup	150	0	0
Wheaties (General Mills)	1 cup	104	1	1

CHEESES

American cheese, processed				
(Velveeta)	1 oz	80	54	68
reduced fat (Kraft)	1 oz	70	36	51
slice	1 oz	95	62	65
American cheese spread, processed	1 oz	80	53	66
Blue cheese	1 oz	103	77	75
Brick cheese	1 oz	105	72	69
Brie cheese	1 oz	95	71	75
Camembert cheese	1 oz	84	62	74
Caraway cheese	1 oz	107	75	70

FOOD		CALORIES		
	AMOUNT	TOTAL	FAT	%FAT
Cheddar cheese	1 oz	112	82	73
food spread with wine (Kraft)	1 oz	90	54	60
food spread sharp (Kraft)	1 oz	90	63	70
grated or shredded	1/2 cup	229	167	73
Light Naturals (Kraft)	1 oz	80	45	56
Cheese ball ✔	1 Tbsp	64	54	84
Cheese fondue ✔	1/4 cup	170	105	62
Cheese sauce ✔	1/4 cup	132	88	67
	1 Tbsp	33	22	67
Cheese spread, processed (Cheez Whiz)	1 oz	80	54	68
Cheese, low-fat (Olympia)	1 oz	87	54	62
Cheezola	1 oz	90	63	70
Cheshire cheese	1 oz	110	77	70
Colby cheese	1 oz	112	82	73
Cottage cheese				
1% fat, all curds	1/2 cup	83	9	11
2% fat, all curds	1/2 cup	103	18	17
4% fat, all curds	1/2 cup	118	44	37
dry curd	1/2 cup	63	5	8
Cream cheese				
Light, Philadelphia	1 oz	60	45	75
Philadelphia	1 oz	100	90	90
Philadelphia, soft tub	2 Tbsp	100	90	90
reduced fat, Neufchatel	1 oz	74	58	78
Edam cheese	1 oz	101	70	69
Farmer's cheese	1 oz	90	63	70
Feta cheese	1 oz	75	53	71
Fontina cheese	1 oz	110	77	70
Gjetost cheese	1 oz	132	74	56
Gouda cheese	1 oz	101	69	68
Green River cheese, part skim milk	1 oz	101	66	65
Gruyere cheese	1 oz	117	81	69
Havarti	1 oz	117	94	80
Jarlsberg	1 oz	100	63	63
Laughing Cow, reduced calorie cheese	1 oz	50	27	54
Light N' Lively cheese (Kraft)	1 oz	70	36	51

FOOD

CALORIES

	AMOUNT	TOTAL	FAT	%FAT
Limburger cheese	1 oz	90	66	73
Lite-Line, 1 1/2 slice = 1 oz	1 oz	50	18	36
low cholesterol	1 oz	90	63	70
Macaroni and Cheese				
(Kraft)	1 cup	363	146	40
canned	1 cup	230	90	39
from mix	1 cup	267	24	9
with 3.8% milk	1 cup	305	198	65
with skim milk	1 cup	281	171	61
Monterey Jack cheese	1 oz	106	76	72
Light Naturals (Kraft)	1 oz	80	45	56
Mozzarella cheese				
Light Naturals (Kraft)	1 oz	80	36	45
part skim	1 oz	72	40	56
whole milk	1 oz	90	62	69
Mozzarella, low moisture, part skim	1 oz	78	43	55
Muenster cheese	1 oz	104	75	72
Neufchatel, reduced fat cream cheese	1 oz	74	58	78
Parmesan cheese, grated	1 Tbsp	25	18	72
	1 oz	120	86	72
	1/2 cup	200	144	72
Pimiento cheese, processed	1 oz	106	80	75
Port du Salut cheese	1 oz	100	72	72
Pot cheese	1 oz	25	tr	tr
Provolone cheese	1 oz	100	70	70
Ricotta cheese				
part skim	1/2 cup	170	84	49
whole milk	1/2 cup	215	141	66
Ricotta, whey, low-fat (Piazza)	1/2 cup	120	36	30
Romano cheese, grated	1 Tbsp	19	11	58
	1 oz	114	66	58
	1/2 cup	152	88	58
Roquefort cheese	1 oz	105	78	74
Swiss cheese	1 oz	105	70	67
Light Naturals (Kraft)	1 oz	90	45	50
reduced fat (Hickory Farm)	1 oz	80	54	68

FOOD		CALORIES		
	AMOUNT	TOTAL	FAT	%FAT
Swiss cheese food, processed	1 oz	95	63	66
Tilsit cheese	1 oz	97	66	68
Welsh rarebit ✔	1/4 cup	295	162	55

CONDIMENTS

Barbecue sauce	1 Tbsp	20	4	20
	1/2 cup	160	32	20
Beets, canned, pickled	1/2 cup	81	tr	tr
Bread and butter pickles ✔	1/4 cup	95	0	0
Catsup	1/2 cup	145	4	3
	1 Tbsp	15	tr	tr
Chicken McNugget sauce (McDonald's)				
barbeque	1 oz	50	5	10
honey	1/2 oz	45	0	0
hot mustard	1 oz	70	32	46
sweet and sour	1 oz	60	2	3
Chili powder	1 tsp	5	tr	tr
Cocktail sauce ✔	1 Tbsp	15	0	0
Cranberry orange relish ✔	1 Tbsp	27	1	4
Cranberry sauce, canned, sweetened	1/4 cup	102	2	2
Curry sauce ✔	1 Tbsp	26	18	69
Dill sauce ✔	1/4 cup	18	9	50
Giblet gravy ✔	1/4 cup	47	9	19
Herb-garlic sauce ✔	1 Tbsp	27	18	67
Hollandaise sauce ✔	1 Tbsp	45	42	93
	1/4 cup	180	167	93
Honey butter ✔	1 Tbsp	60	48	80
Horseradish sauce, creamy (Kraft)	1 Tbsp	50	45	90
Horseradish, prepared	1 Tbsp	7	tr	tr
Hummus ✔	1/4 cup	105	47	45
Jalapeno peppers, chopped	1/2 cup	17	tr	tr

FOOD		CALORIES		
	AMOUNT	TOTAL	FAT	%FAT
Molly McButter, all flavors	1 tsp	8	0	0
Mustard				
dry	1 tsp	12	8	67
with horseradish	1 tsp	4	2	50
yellow	1 tsp	5	tr	tr
Olives				
black, ripe, extra large	1 olive	9	8	89
sliced	1 cup	174	155	89
Greek	1 olive	7	6	86
green, large, 1" diameter	1 olive	5	4	80
small	1 olive	3	3	100
Onion dip ✔	1 Tbsp	55	54	98
Pesto, basil ✔	1 Tbsp	123	117	95
Pickle relish				
sour	1 Tbsp	3	tr	tr
sweet	1 Tbsp	20	tr	tr
Pickled beets, canned	1/2 cup	55	tr	tr
Pickles				
dill, medium, whole	1 pickle	5	tr	tr
sweet gherkins, whole	1 pickle	20	tr	tr
Rice vinegar				
regular (Marukan)	1 Tbsp	1	0	0
seasoned (Marukan)	1 Tbsp	30	0	0
Shake 'n Bake mix	1 oz	116	38	33
Soy sauce, regular or lite	1 Tbsp	10	tr	tr
Spaghetti sauce				
with meat ✔	1 cup	297	167	56
without meat ✔	1 cup	171	72	42
meat flavored				
(Prego)	1 cup	288	72	25
(Ragú)	1 cup	160	36	23
plain (Ragú)	1 cup	160	54	34
plain or mushroom (Prego)	1 cup	276	72	26
Sweet-sour sauce ✔	1/4 cup	99	0	0
Tabasco pepper sauce	1/4 tsp	tr	tr	tr
Taco sauce	1/2 cup	28	2	7

FOOD

CALORIES

	AMOUNT	TOTAL	FAT	%FAT
Tartar sauce, regular	1 Tbsp	75	72	96
Teriyaki sauce	1 Tbsp	17	tr	tr
Tomato catsup	1 Tbsp	15	tr	tr
	1/2 cup	145	4	3
Tomato paste	1 Tbsp	12	tr	tr
	1/2 cup	96	tr	tr
Tomato puree	1/2 cup	49	2	4
	1 Tbsp	6	tr	tr
Tomato sauce, regular or Spanish	1/2 cup	43	3	7
	1 Tbsp	5	tr	tr
Vinegar				
cider or white distilled	1 Tbsp	tr	tr	tr
rice, regular (Marukan)	1 Tbsp	1	0	0
rice, seasoned (Marukan)	1 Tbsp	30	0	0
White sauce, medium ✔	1 Tbsp	27	18	67
	1/4 cup	107	73	68
Worcestershire sauce	1 tsp	4	0	0

COOKIES

	AMOUNT	TOTAL	FAT	%FAT
Almond cookie, Chinese, 2" diameter	1 cookie	153	97	63
Animal crackers	5 pieces	43	8	19
Arrowroot cookie (Nabisco)	1 cookie	23	7	30
Brownie, fudge				
1/24 mix (Betty Crocker)	1 brownie	130	45	35
mix (Betty Crocker)	1 mix	3120	1080	35
with walnuts, 1/24 mix (Betty Crocker)	1 brownie	160	63	39
with walnuts, mix (Betty Crocker)	1 mix	3840	1512	39
Brownie, chocolate, plain, 2" square ✔	1 brownie	146	85	58
Butter cookie, spritz	1 cookie	23	8	35

FOOD

CALORIES

	AMOUNT	TOTAL	FAT	%FAT
Chocolate chip cookie				
3" diameter	1 cookie	65	32	49
Almost Home (Nabisco)	1 cookie	60	27	45
Big Batch mix	1 cookie	120	54	45
Big Batch, 36 cookies	1 pkg	4320	1944	45
commercial, 1 3/4" diameter	1 small	34	14	41
(Dunkin' Donuts)	1 cookie	129	63	49
(McDonald's)	1 box	330	140	43
(Wendy's)	1 cookie	320	153	48
Cookie dough, plain, chilled roll, 18 oz	1 roll	2290	1037	45
Fig bar cookie, 1 5/8 x 3/8" square	1 cookie	50	6	12
Fortune cookie, Chinese	1 cookie	66	36	55
Gingersnap cookie, 3" diameter	1 cookie	34	6	18
Graham cracker	1 square	30	5	16
chocolate covered	1 square	60	27	45
snacks, Teddy Grahams, 11=1/2 oz	1/2 oz	60	18	30
Granola bar (Nature Valley)				
chewey	1 bar	140	63	45
plain	1 bar	110	36	33
with fruit	1 bar	150	45	30
Ice cream cone, plain, without ice cream	1 cone	18	2	11
sugar, without ice cream	1 cone	49	39	80
waffle, without ice cream	1 average	118	25	21
Jam thumbprints ✔	1 cookie	84	45	54
Macaroon cookie, 3" diameter	1 cookie	98	41	42
(Dunkin' Donuts)	1 cookie	351	171	49
Marshmallow cookie, with coconut or chocolate topping	1 cookie	74	22	30
McDonaldland cookies (McDonald's)	1 box	290	83	29
Oatmeal cookie				
homemade ✔	1 cookie	80	29	36
Big Batch mix	1 cookie	130	54	42
Big Batch mix, 36 cookies	1 pkg	4680	1944	42
with raisins, 3" diameter	1 cookie	82	25	30
Oreo cookie (Nabisco)	1 cookie	40	18	45
Peanut butter cookie, 3" diameter ✔	1 cookie	91	45	49

FOOD

CALORIES

	AMOUNT	TOTAL	FAT	%FAT
Peanut butter oatmeal bars ✔	1 bar	116	54	47
Peanut butter sandwich cookie, 1 3/4" diameter	1 cookie	58	21	36
Sandwich type cookie, chocolate or vanilla	1 cookie	50	19	38
Shortbread cookie, 1 5/8" square x 1/4"	1 cookie	37	16	43
Snickerdoodles ✔	1 cookie	79	27	34
Spritz ✔	1 cookie	81	45	56
Strawberry Newtons (Nabisco)	1 cookie	80	18	23
Sugar cookie, 3" diameter ✔	1 cookie	48	21	44
Vanilla wafer cookie, 1 3/4" diameter	1 cookie	18	5	28

CRACKERS AND CHIPS

	AMOUNT	TOTAL	FAT	%FAT
Animal crackers	5 crackers	43	8	19
Apple chips	1 oz	120	45	38
Better Cheddars (Nabisco)	1 cracker	6	3	50
Bread sticks, hard, 7x1/2"	1 stick	27	2	7
Cereal party mix	1 cup	418	261	62
Chee-tos, cheese flavor snack, 57 = 1 3/4 oz	1 3/4 oz	280	153	55
Cheez-It (Sunshine)	1 cracker	6	3	50
Cheese puffs, snack food, 25 = 1 cup	1 cup	96	54	56
Chicken in a Biscuit (Nabisco)	1 cracker	10	5	50
Corn chips				
10 chips = 1 oz (Tostitos)	1 oz	150	72	48
15 chips = 1 oz (Doritos)	1 oz	140	56	40
15 chips = 1 oz (Frito Lay	1 oz	160	90	56
Corn nuts, snack food	1 oz	110	27	25
Cracked wheat crackers (Pepperidge Farm)	1 cracker	28	9	32
Cracklebred (Jacquet)	1 cracker	17	tr	tr

FOOD

CALORIES

	AMOUNT	TOTAL	FAT	%FAT
Crispbread, High Fiber (Ryvita)	1 cracker	23	tr	tr
Doo Dads snack mix	1/2 cup	140	54	39
English Water Biscuit (Pepperidge Farm)	1 cracker	18	2	11
Goldfish crackers (Pepperidge Farm)	1 oz	136	51	38
Graham cracker	1 square	30	5	16
chocolate covered	1 square	60	27	45
Graham cracker crumbs	1 Tbsp	29	6	21
	1 cup	462	98	21
Hearty Wheat crackers (Pepperidge Farm)	1 cracker	25	16	64
Hi-Ho Deluxe crackers (Sunshine)	1 cracker	20	11	55
Matzoh cracker	1 piece	117	3	3
Melba toast, plain	1 slice	15	2	13
Norwegian flat bread (Kavli)	1 wafer	35	0	0
Oriental party mix	1 oz	150	81	54
Oyster crackers	10 cracker	43	10	23
Peanut Butter 'n Cheese (Handi-Snacks)	1 pkg	190	117	62
Potato chips				
45 = 1 1/8 oz (Frito Lay)	1 1/8 oz	170	99	58
Bar-B-Que (Frito Lay)	1 oz	150	81	54
O'Grady, 1 oz (Frito Lay)	8 chips	150	81	54
(Pringle's)	1 oz	170	117	69
Ruffles, 25 = 1 1/8 oz (Frito Lay)	1 1/8 oz	170	90	53
Sour Cream and Onion (Frito Lay)	1 oz	160	90	56
Pretzels				
Dutch, 28 per lb	1 large	58	2	3
soft	1 pretzel	158	27	17
three ring, 148 per lb	1 piece	12	1	8
very thin sticks, 1600 per lb	1 piece	10	tr	tr
Rice cakes	1 cake	35	3	9
mini	1 cake	12	tr	tr
Ritz cracker	1 cracker	18	8	44
Ry-Krisp cracker, natural	1 triple	22	1	5
Rye wafers, whole grain	1 wafer	23	tr	tr
Saltine crackers, 2" square	2 crackers	25	4	16
Soy nuts, snack food	1 cup	63	24	38

FOOD		CALORIES		
	AMOUNT	TOTAL	FAT	%FAT
Taco chips, 10 chips = 1 oz (Tostitos)	1 oz	140	72	51
Town House crackers (Keebler)	1 cracker	17	9	53
Triscuit cracker (Nabisco)	1 cracker	21	13	62
Wasa crisp bread, Hearty Rye	1 cracker	45	tr	tr
Lite Rye	1 cracker	25	tr	tr
Sesame Wheat	1 cracker	50	18	36
Wheat Thin cracker (Nabisco)	1 cracker	9	3	33
Cheese	1 cracker	8	3	38
Nutty	1 cracker	11	6	55
Wheatsworth cracker (Nabisco)	1 cracker	14	6	43

Dairy and Non-Dairy Products

	AMOUNT	TOTAL	FAT	%FAT
Buttermilk				
cultured, powder, reconstituted	1 cup	79	6	8
dried	1/2 cup	233	31	13
skim	1 cup	88	2	2
Chocolate milk				
1%	1 cup	160	26	16
2%, lowfat	1 cup	180	45	25
3.8%, whole	1 cup	210	72	34
Cool Whip topping	1 Tbsp	12	9	75
	1 cup	192	144	75
Extra Creamy	1 Tbsp	16	11	69
	1 cup	256	176	69
Lite	1 Tbsp	8	6	75
	1 cup	128	96	75

FOOD		CALORIES		
	AMOUNT	TOTAL	FAT	%FAT
Cream				
half-and-half	1 Tbsp	20	17	85
	1 cup	320	272	85
light	1 Tbsp	30	28	93
	1 cup	480	448	93
whipping, heavy, unwhipped	1 Tbsp	53	50	94
	1 cup	848	800	94
whipped	1 Tbsp	26	25	96
	1 cup	416	400	96
Creamer, dry				
Coffee Mate (Carnation)	1 Tbsp	30	27	90
Lite	1 Tbsp	24	18	75
Cremora (Borden)	1 Tbsp	36	27	75
Creamer, imitation, liquid				
(Carnation)	1 Tbsp	33	18	55
(Mocha Mix)	1 Tbsp	20	18	90
Eggnog (nonalcoholic)	1 cup	340	171	50
Evaporated milk, skim	1 cup	200	9	5
whole	1 cup	340	171	50
Half-and-half, cream	1 Tbsp	20	17	85
	1 cup	320	272	85
I.M.O., imitation sour cream	1 Tbsp	30	27	90
	1 cup	480	432	90
Instant Breakfast, with 3.8% milk (Carnation)	1 cup	280	81	29
Le Creme topping	1 Tbsp	12	9	75
	1 cup	192	144	75
Malted milk, made with 3.8% milk	1 cup	236	89	38
Milk				
chocolate				
1%	1 cup	160	26	16
2%, lowfat	1 cup	180	45	25
3.8%, whole	1 cup	210	72	34
skim	1 cup	85	tr	tr
1%	1 cup	102	24	24
2%, lowfat	1 cup	122	42	34
3.8%, whole	1 cup	161	81	50

FOOD

CALORIES

	AMOUNT	TOTAL	FAT	%FAT
Milk, condensed, sweetened	1 cup	980	243	25
Milk, goat	1 cup	163	88	54
Milk, instant nonfat dry	1 cup	245	tr	tr
reconstituted	1 cup	81	tr	tr
Milk, skim, evaporated, unsweetened	1 cup	200	9	5
Milk, whole, evaporated, unsweetened	1 cup	340	171	50
Ovaltine, malt or chocolate powder	3/4 oz	78	8	10
Skim milk	1 cup	85	tr	tr
Sour cream	1 Tbsp	31	27	87
	1 cup	495	432	87
Sour cream, half-and-half	1 Tbsp	21	16	76
	1 cup	335	251	75
Soy milk	1 cup	79	45	57
Sweetened condensed milk, canned	1 cup	980	243	25
Yogurt (Yoplait)				
breakfast style	6 oz	220	27	12
custard style	6 oz	190	36	19
fruit flavors, light	6 oz	90	5	6
plain	6 oz	120	27	23
Yogurt, low-fat				
fruit-flavored	1 cup	240	27	11
plain	1 Tbsp	9	2	22
	1 cup	140	31	22
vanilla, lemon or coffee	1 cup	200	27	14
Yogurt, non-fat				
plain	1 cup	110	tr	tr
with fruit	1 cup	150	tr	tr
Yogurt, whole milk	1 cup	150	63	42

FOOD

CALORIES

	AMOUNT	TOTAL	FAT	%FAT
DONUTS AND PASTRIES				
Apple brown betty ✔	1/2 cup	211	44	21
Apple crisp ✔	1/2 cup	302	73	24
Apple dumplings ✔	1 cup	755	297	39
Apple fritters (Mrs. Paul's)	1 piece	120	53	44
Apple strudel, frozen (Pepperidge Farm)	1 serving	290	129	44
Babka, 8" diameter	1 roll	1361	926	68
Baklava, walnut, 1 x 2" piece	1 piece	117	55	47
Blintz, cheese, fruit filled, 6"	1 blintz	164	33	20
Cinnamon roll, plain, small, 3" diameter				
(Pillsbury)	1 roll	145	56	39
homemade ✔	1 roll	176	45	26
Coffeecake, 2 3/4" square	1 piece	230	62	27
8 x 5 1/2 x 1 1/4"	1 cake	1385	361	26
Cream puff, shell, 3 1/2 x 2" ✔	1 shell	156	105	67
with custard filling	1 average	303	163	54
with whipped cream filling ✔	1 average	279	216	77
Crepes suzette ✔	2 crepes	334	144	43
Cupcake, plain, from mix, 2 1/2" diameter	1 cupcake	88	27	31
Danish				
apple, frozen (Sara Lee)	1 roll	360	122	34
caramel, refrigerated (Pillsbury)	1 roll	157	68	43
cheese, frozen (Sara Lee)	1 roll	308	151	49
Ding dong, 1 1/2" diameter (Hostess)	1 piece	187	95	51
Donut, cake, iced or sugared,				
3 1/4" diameter	1 average	184	71	39
Donut, plain				
1 1/2" diameter	1 donut	55	23	42
2 1/2" diameter	1 donut	98	41	42
3 1/4" diameter	1 donut	164	69	42
3 5/8" diameter	1 donut	227	95	42
Donut, raised or yeast				
plain, 3 1/4" diameter	1 average	174	100	57
jelly, 3 1/2" diameter	1 average	226	79	35
cream filled, 3 1/2" diameter	1 average	244	85	35

FOOD	AMOUNT	CALORIES		
		TOTAL	FAT	%FAT
Eclair				
with custard filling and chocolate icing	1 average	263	135	51
with pudding ✔	1 average	290	135	47
Flan	1/2 cup	180	79	44
Hot cross buns	1 average	111	29	26
Maple bar, or Long John, 5 x 2"	1 piece	324	179	55
Rosettes, 2 1/2" diameter ✔	1 average	33	14	42
Snowball, 2" diameter (Hostess)	1 piece	160	45	28
Sopaipillas, 3" x 3"	1 piece	141	107	76
Sweet roll, commercial, 2 oz	1 roll	178	38	21
Turnover				
apple, 3 oz	1 turnover	255	127	50
cherry, 3 oz	1 turnover	251	127	51
lemon, 3 oz	1 turnover	279	137	49
Twinkie, 3 x 3/4" (Hostess)	1 piece	163	54	33

EGGS

Cheese omelet ✔	2 eggs	379	288	76
Egg and sausage casserole ✔	1 cup	663	495	75
Egg McMuffin (McDonald's)	1 serving	290	101	35
Egg salad ✔	1/2 cup	307	249	81
Egg substitute (Second Nature)	1/4 cup	53	24	45
frozen (Egg Beaters)	1/4 cup	25	0	0
(Morning Star Farms)	1/4 cup	60	27	45

FOOD

CALORIES

	AMOUNT	TOTAL	FAT	%FAT
Egg				
hard/soft boiled, without fat	1 egg	75	45	60
omelet, plain, 2 eggs	1 serving	189	128	68
poached, without fat	1 egg	75	45	60
poached/fried with 1 tsp fat	1 egg	109	79	72
Egg, raw, large				
white	1 white	17	tr	tr
whole	1 egg	75	45	60
yolk	1 yolk	58	45	78
Egg, turkey, raw, whole	1 medium	135	85	63
Eggs Benedict ✔	1 serving	465	324	70
Eggs, deviled ✔	2 halves	145	116	80
Eggs, scrambled (McDonald's)	1 serving	140	88	63
Huevos rancheros ✔	1 egg	466	25	5
Omelet, French ✔	2 eggs	266	207	78
Quiche Lorraine, 1/6 of 9" pie ✔	1 piece	543	351	65
Vegetable Omelet mix (Egg Beaters)	1/4 cup	27	0	0

ENTREES

	AMOUNT	TOTAL	FAT	%FAT
Arroz con Pollo, with 1/2 cup rice ✔	4 oz meat	403	90	22
Beef and vegetable stir-fry, with rice ✔	1 1/2 cups	513	189	37
Beef kebabs ✔	1 kebab	358	207	58
Beef potpie, 4 1/4" diameter ✔	1 pie	558	296	53
Beef stew				
canned (Nalley)	1 cup	190	54	28
homemade ✔	1 cup	225	77	34
Beef stroganoff, with noodles ✔	1 1/2 cups	735	495	67
Beefaroni (Chef Boyardee)	1 cup	213	54	25
Bouillabaisse ✔	1 cup	245	84	34

FOOD		CALORIES		
	AMOUNT	TOTAL	FAT	%FAT
Burrito				
bean and cheese, 5 oz	1 burrito	339	99	29
beef and bean, 5 oz	1 burrito	366	135	37
green chili, 5 oz	1 burrito	353	117	33
red hot beef, 5 oz	1 burrito	319	109	34
Cabbage rolls, stuffed with ground beef	1 medium	193	95	49
Cannelloni ✔	1 each	134	45	34
Chicken 'a la King ✔	1 cup	233	121	52
over 1/2 English muffin	1 cup sauce	313	130	42
Chicken and dumplings, with 1 dumpling	3 oz meat	255	81	32
Chicken Cacciatore, 1/2 breast	1 serving	235	126	54
with 1/2 cup rice ✔	4 oz meat	327	99	30
Chicken, curried with 3/4 cup vegetables	4 oz meat	462	171	37
Chicken, fried ✔	4 oz meat	218	99	45
Chicken divan ✔	1 cup	337	189	56
Chicken enchiladas ✔	2 each	535	279	52
Chicken fricassee ✔	4 oz meat	376	135	36
Chicken Kiev ✔	4 oz meat	334	171	51
Chicken livers, with tomato sauce and noodles	3 oz meat	351	108	31
Chicken parmesan ✔	4 oz meat	290	144	50
Chicken pot pie, 5" diameter ✔	1 pie	619	315	51
Chicken stew (Chef Boyardee)	1 cup	160	54	34
Chicken teriyaki kebabs ✔	1 kebab	194	36	19
Chicken, stewed	4 oz meat	167	54	32
Chili (Wendy's)	1 cup	230	81	35
Chili con carne, homemade ✔	1 cup	481	225	47
with beans, canned (Stokley)	1 cup	390	234	60
without beans, canned (Stokley)	1 cup	430	315	73
Chili with beans, lite (Dennison's)	1 cup	213	45	21
Chili, chicken, with beans, lite (Dennison's)	1 cup	224	45	20
Chili, meatless ✔	1 cup	260	28	11
Chipped beef, creamed ✔	1 cup	357	228	64
with 3.8% milk ✔	1 cup	274	135	49
with skim milk ✔	1 cup	243	104	43
Coney Island ✔	1 serving	373	225	60

FOOD		CALORIES		
	AMOUNT	TOTAL	FAT	%FAT
Corn dog	1 serving	345	202	59
Crab cocktail	2 oz	52	9	17
Crab stuffed chicken breasts ✔	1/2 breast	449	135	30
Crepe, without filling, 6" diameter	1 crepe	58	24	41
with shrimp filling (Mrs. Smith's)	2 crepes	305	144	47
Dim Sum, 4 oz ✔	1 roll	345	189	55
Eggplant parmigiana ✔	1 cup	336	155	46
Fettucini Alfredo ✔	1 cup	550	306	57
Fish Creole ✔	4 oz fish	351	108	31
Fish Florentine ✔	4 oz fish	240	108	45
Gnocchi, cheese, baked ✔	1 cup	449	261	58
Ham-noodle casserole ✔	1 cup	513	288	56
Hasenpfeffer ✔	4 oz	371	144	39
Jambalaya, shrimp ✔	1 cup	450	153	34
Lasagna, 4 x 3 x 2" ✔	1 piece	633	396	63
Lima Beans with Ham (Dennison's)	1 cup	267	63	24
Liver and onions ✔	4 oz liver	318	163	51
Lobster tail, grilled, with butter	5 oz	232	117	50
Macaroni and Cheese				
(Kraft)	1 cup	363	146	40
canned	1 cup	230	90	39
from mix	1 cup	267	24	9
with 3.8% milk ✔	1 cup	305	198	65
with skim milk ✔	1 cup	281	171	61
Manicotti, stuffed ✔	1 each	188	54	29
Meat loaf, 1 1/2 x 4 x 2" ✔	1 slice	417	243	58
all beef ✔	1 oz	51	20	39
with beef and pork ✔	1 oz	53	22	42
Meatballs with tomato sauce ✔	1 cup	209	136	65
Moo goo gai pan ✔	1 cup	566	307	54
Oysters Rockefeller ✔	6 oysters	200	99	50
Pepper, stuffed, 2 3/4" long ✔	1 pepper	322	167	52
Pierogies, 1 3/4 x 1 3/4" ✔	1 piece	75	35	47
Pizza, deep dish, cheese/tomato,				
5 1/4 x 3 3/4"	1 slice	421	122	29

FOOD | CALORIES

	AMOUNT	TOTAL	FAT	%FAT
Pizza, 1/8 of 16" diameter (Domino's)				
cheese	1 slice	188	45	24
deluxe	1 slice	249	92	37
double cheese, pepperoni	1 slice	273	114	42
ham, Canadian-style	1 slice	209	50	24
pepperoni	1 slice	230	79	34
sausage, mushroom	1 slice	215	71	33
veggie	1 slice	249	83	34
Pizza, Thin 'n Crispy, 15" (Pizza Hut)				
cheese	1 pizza	1592	616	38
pepperoni	1 pizza	1656	720	43
supreme	1 pizza	1840	792	43
super supreme	1 pizza	1856	760	41
Pork chow mein, with rice ✔	1 1/2 cups	464	234	50
Pot pie, beef, 4 1/4" diameter ✔	1 pie	558	296	53
Potato-ham scallop ✔	1 1/4 cups	540	207	38
Quesadilla ✔	5 oz	739	429	58
Quiche Lorraine, 1/6 of 9" pie ✔	1 piece	543	351	65
Quiche, seafood, 1/6 of 9" pie ✔	1 piece	496	297	60
Ravioli, canned	1 cup	256	72	28
homemade, with meat filling ✔	1 cup	323	113	35
Salisbury steak ✔	5 oz	596	378	63
Salmon loaf, 2 x 2 x 3" ✔	1 slice	341	135	40
Scallopini, veal	1 cup	790	359	45
Shrimp chow mein ✔	1 1/2 cups	455	153	34
Shrimp crepes (Mrs. Smith's)	2 crepes	305	144	47
Shrimp Newburg ✔	1 cup	572	387	68
Sloppy Joe mixture, without roll	1 cup	568	343	60
Spaghetti sauce				
with meat ✔	1 cup	297	167	56
without meat ✔	1 cup	171	72	42
meat flavored (Prego)	1 cup	288	72	25
(Ragú)	1 cup	160	36	23
plain (Ragú)	1 cup	160	54	34
plain or mushroom (Prego)	1 cup	276	72	26
Spaghetti with meat balls ✔	1 cup	332	105	32

FOOD		CALORIES		
	AMOUNT	TOTAL	FAT	%FAT
Stewed chicken ✔	4 oz meat	167	54	32
Stroganoff, beef, with noodles ✔	1 1/2 cups	735	495	67
Stuffed cabbage rolls ✔	1 roll	314	180	57
Stuffed cornish game hens ✔	1/2 hen	385	216	56
Stuffed flounder ✔	4 oz fish	311	153	49
Stuffed manicotti ✔	1 each	188	54	29
Stuffed pepper, 2 3/4" long ✔	1 pepper	322	167	52
Stuffed pork chops ✔	1 chop	802	585	73
Sushi over 1/4 cup rice	1 cup	250	6	2
Sweet and sour pork, Chinese	1 cup	344	209	61
Swiss steak, 3 x 3 x 1/2" ✔	1 piece	214	81	38
Tempura ✔	1 cup	264	209	79
Tetrazzini, chicken	1 cup	442	185	42
Tortellini, cooked				
cheese	1 cup	754	108	14
meat	1 cup	754	108	14
Trout Amandine ✔	4 oz fish	264	180	68
Tuna-noodle casserole ✔	1 cup	393	168	43
Veal parmigiana ✔	4 oz meat	408	248	61
Veal scallopini ✔	4 oz meat	387	204	53
Vegetable stir-fry, meatless ✔	1 cup	94	45	48

FAST FOODS

Arby's

Beef 'n cheddar sandwich	1 sandwich	455	241	53
Chicken breast sandwich	1 sandwich	493	225	46

FOOD

CALORIES

	AMOUNT	TOTAL	FAT	%FAT
Chicken club sandwich	1 sandwich	610	297	49
French fries, 2.5 oz	1 serving	246	119	48
Ham 'n cheese sandwich	1 sandwich	292	123	42
Jamocha shake, 11.5 oz	1 shake	368	95	26
Potato cakes, 3 oz	1 serving	204	108	53
Roast beef sandwich, regular	1 sandwich	353	133	38
Super	1 serving	501	199	40
Turkey deluxe sandwich	1 sandwich	375	149	40

Burger King

	AMOUNT	TOTAL	FAT	%FAT
Apple pie	1 serving	305	108	35
Bagel sandwich, breakfast	1 sandwich	387	126	33
BK Broiler	1 sandwich	379	162	43
Cheeseburger	1 burger	317	135	43
Cheeseburger, bacon, double	1 burger	510	279	55
Cheesburger deluxe	1 burger	364	180	49
Chicken specialty sandwich	1 sandwich	688	360	52
Chicken tenders	1 serving	204	90	44
Croissanwich, breakfast				
bacon	1 sandwich	355	216	61
ham	1 sandwich	335	180	54
sausage	1 sandwich	538	369	69
Danish, great	1 roll	500	324	65
French fries, regular	1 serving	227	117	52
French toast sticks	1 serving	499	261	52
Ham and cheese specialty sandwich	1 sandwich	471	207	44
Hamburger	1 burger	275	108	39
Hamburger deluxe	1 burger	322	153	48
Milkshake				
chocolate	1 shake	320	108	34
vanilla	1 shake	321	90	28
Onion rings	1 serving	274	144	53
Salad				
Chef	1 salad	180	81	45
Chicken	1 salad	140	36	26
Garden	1 salad	90	45	50

FOOD		CALORIES		
	AMOUNT	TOTAL	FAT	%FAT
Salad dressing				
Blue cheese	1 packet	300	279	93
French	1 packet	280	207	74
House	1 packet	260	234	90
Italian, reduced calorie	1 packet	30	18	60
Thousand Island	1 packet	240	207	86
Whaler fish sandwich	1 sandwich	488	243	50
Whopper	1 burger	628	324	52
with cheese	1 burger	711	387	54
Dairy Queen				
Banana split	1 serving	540	99	18
Blizzard, 16 oz				
Butterfinger	1 serving	765	252	33
Hawaiian	1 serving	700	198	28
Heath	1 serving	800	216	27
Strawberry	1 serving	675	153	23
Buster bar	1 serving	460	261	57
Cheeseburger				
double	1 burger	650	333	51
single	1 burger	410	180	44
triple	1 burger	820	450	55
Chicken sandwich	1 sandwich	670	369	55
Dilly bar	1 serving	210	117	56
DQ sandwich	1 sandwich	140	36	26
Fish sandwich	1 sandwich	400	153	38
with cheese	1 sandwich	440	189	43
French fries				
large	1 serving	320	144	45
regular	1 serving	200	90	45
Float	1 serving	410	63	15

FOOD

CALORIES

	AMOUNT	TOTAL	FAT	%FAT
Freeze	1 serving	500	108	22
Hamburger				
double	1 burger	530	252	48
single	1 burger	360	144	40
triple	1 burger	710	405	57
Hot dog				
cheese	1 serving	330	189	57
chili	1 serving	320	180	56
regular	1 serving	280	144	51
super	1 serving	520	243	47
Hot fudge brownie delight	1 serving	600	225	38
Malt				
large	1 malt	1060	225	21
regular	1 malt	760	162	21
small	1 malt	520	108	21
Milkshake				
large	1 shake	990	234	24
regular	1 shake	710	171	24
small	1 shake	490	117	24
Mr. Misty				
float	1 serving	390	63	16
freeze	1 serving	500	108	22
kiss	1 serving	70	0	0
Parfait	1 serving	430	72	17
double delight	1 serving	490	180	37
peanut buster	1 serving	740	306	41
Soft serve ice cream without cone	1 cup	261	78	30
Soft serve ice cream with cone				
large	1 cone	340	90	26
regular	1 cone	240	63	26
small	1 cone	140	36	26
Soft serve ice cream with cone, dipped				
large	1 cone	510	216	42
regular	1 cone	340	144	42
small	1 cone	190	80	42

FOOD

CALORIES

	AMOUNT	TOTAL	FAT	%FAT
Sundae, all varieties				
large	1 serving	440	90	20
regular	1 serving	310	72	23
small	1 serving	190	36	19
Dunkin' Donuts				
Biscuit	1 biscuit	332	207	62
Brownie	1 brownie	280	117	42
Chocolate chip cookie	1 cookie	129	63	49
Croissant				
almond	1 croissant	435	270	62
chocolate	1 croissant	502	333	66
plain	1 croissant	291	198	68
Donut				
apple filled with cinnamon sugar	1 donut	219	108	49
Bavarian creme filled	1 donut	226	126	56
Bavarian filled with chocolate frosting	1 donut	231	81	35
blueberry filled	1 donut	196	90	46
chocolate cake ring with glaze	1 donut	324	189	58
chocolate frosted yeast ring	1 donut	246	126	51
coconut coated cake ring	1 donut	417	252	60
French cruller with glaze	1 donut	201	126	63
honey dipped coffee roll	1 donut	348	153	44
honey dipped cruller	1 donut	370	207	56
honey dipped yeast ring	1 donut	208	99	48
jelly filled	1 donut	274	198	72
lemon filled	1 donut	221	99	45
Munchkin cake with powdered sugar	1 donut	69	36	52
Munchkin chocolate with glaze	1 donut	88	45	51
Munchkin yeast with glaze	1 donut	43	18	42
plain cake ring	1 donut	319	198	62
sugar jelly stick	1 donut	332	162	49

FOOD		CALORIES		
	AMOUNT	TOTAL	FAT	%FAT
Macaroon	1 cookie	351	171	49
Muffins				
apple spice	1 muffin	327	99	30
banana nut	1 muffin	327	108	33
blueberry	1 muffin	263	90	34
bran	1 muffin	353	117	33
cherry	1 muffin	317	90	28
corn	1 muffin	347	117	34
Hardee's				
Big Country breakfast with ham	1 serving	620	297	48
Big Twin	1 burger	450	225	50
Biscuit				
bacon, egg, and cheese	1 biscuit	460	252	55
Canadian Rise 'N Shine	1 biscuit	470	243	52
chicken	1 biscuit	430	198	46
sausage	1 biscuit	440	252	57
sausage and egg	1 biscuit	490	279	57
steak	1 biscuit	500	261	52
Chicken fillet	1 sandwich	370	117	32
Crispy Curls	1 serving	300	144	48
Fisherman's fillet	1 sandwich	500	216	43
French fries, regular	1 serving	230	99	43
Grilled chicken sandwich	1 sandwich	310	81	26
Hash Rounds	1 serving	230	126	55
Hot ham 'n cheese	1 sandwich	330	108	33
Milkshake, chocolate	1 shake	460	72	16
Mushroom 'n Swiss burger	1 burger	490	243	50
Roast beef sandwich				
big	1 sandwich	300	99	33
regular	1 sandwich	260	81	31

FOOD

CALORIES

	AMOUNT	TOTAL	FAT	%FAT
Salad				
Chef	1 salad	240	135	56
Chicken 'n pasta	1 salad	230	27	12
Garden	1 salad	210	126	60
Side	1 salad	20	tr	tr
Turkey club	1 sandwich	390	144	37

Kentucky Fried Chicken

	AMOUNT	TOTAL	FAT	%FAT
Buttermilk biscuits	1 biscuit	232	107	46
Chicken Littles sandwich	1 sandwich	169	90	53
Chicken, extra crispy				
breast	1 piece	354	213	60
drumstick	1 piece	173	98	57
thigh	1 piece	371	234	63
wing	1 piece	218	140	64
Chicken, original recipe				
breast	1 piece	283	135	48
drumstick	1 piece	146	77	52
thigh	1 piece	294	177	60
wing	1 piece	178	105	59
Chicken nuggets	1 piece	46	26	56
Chicken nuggets sauce				
barbeque	1 oz	35	5	14
honey	1/2 oz	49	tr	tr
mustard	1 oz	36	8	22
sweet and sour	1 oz	58	5	9
Coleslaw	1 serving	119	59	50
Corn on the cob	1 piece	176	28	16
French fries	1 serving	244	107	44
Mashed potatoes and gravy	1 serving	71	14	20
Roll	1 roll	61	8	13

FOOD | CALORIES

	AMOUNT	TOTAL	FAT	%FAT
McDonald's				
Apple pie, 3 1/2 oz	1 serving	260	133	51
Big Mac	1 burger	560	292	52
Biscuit				
with bacon, egg and cheese	1 biscuit	440	238	54
with sausage	1 biscuit	440	261	59
with sausage and egg	1 biscuit	520	311	60
with spread	1 biscuit	260	114	44
Cheeseburger	1 burger	310	124	40
Chicken McNuggets, 4 oz	1 serving	290	147	50
Chicken McNugget Sauce				
barbecue	1 oz	50	5	10
honey	1/2 oz	45	0	0
hot mustard	1 oz	70	32	46
sweet and sour	1 oz	60	2	3
Cookies				
chocolate chip	1 box	330	140	43
McDonaldland	1 box	290	83	29
Danish				
apple	1 roll	390	161	41
cinnamon raisin	1 roll	440	189	43
Iced cheese	1 roll	390	196	50
raspberry	1 roll	410	143	35
Egg McMuffin	1 serving	290	101	35
Eggs, scrambled	1 serving	140	88	63
English muffin with butter	1 muffin	170	41	24
Filet-o-fish sandwich	1 sandwich	440	235	53
French fries				
large	1 serving	400	194	49
regular	1 serving	320	154	48
small	1 serving	220	108	49

FOOD		CALORIES		
	AMOUNT	TOTAL	FAT	%FAT
Hamburger	1 burger	260	86	33
Hashbrown potatoes	1 serving	130	66	51
Hotcakes with butter and syrup	1 serving	410	83	20
McChicken sandwich	1 sandwich	490	257	53
McDLT sandwich	1 burger	580	331	57
McMuffin				
sausage	1 serving	370	197	53
sausage with egg	1 serving	440	241	55
Milkshake, 10 oz = 1 shake				
chocolate	1 shake	390	95	24
strawberry	1 shake	380	91	24
vanilla	1 shake	350	92	26
Quarter Pounder	1 burger	410	186	45
with cheese	1 burger	520	263	51
Salad				
Chef	1 salad	230	120	52
Chunky chicken	1 salad	140	31	22
Garden	1 salad	110	59	54
Side	1 salad	60	30	50
Salad dressing				
Blue cheese	1 packet	350	311	89
Caesar	1 packet	300	275	92
French	1 packet	230	187	81
Peppercorn	1 packet	400	392	98
Ranch	1 packet	330	310	94
Red French	1 packet	160	68	43
Thousand Island	1 packet	390	338	87
Vinaigrette, Lite	1 packet	60	18	30
Sausage, pork, 2 oz	1 serving	180	147	82
Soft serve ice cream cone	1 cone	140	41	29
Sundae				
hot caramel	1 sundae	340	82	24
hot fudge	1 sundae	310	85	27
strawberry	1 sundae	280	66	23

FOOD | CALORIES

	AMOUNT	TOTAL	FAT	%FAT
Pizza Hut				
Pan pizza, 1/8 of 14", medium				
cheese	1 slice	246	81	33
pepperoni	1 slice	270	99	37
supreme	1 slice	295	135	46
super supreme	1 slice	282	117	41
Personal pan pizza, 4 1/2" diameter				
pepperoni	1 pizza	338	131	39
supreme	1 pizza	324	126	39
Thin 'n Crispy pizza, 1/8 of 15", medium				
cheese	1 slice	199	77	38
pepperoni	1 slice	207	90	43
supreme	1 slice	230	99	43
super supreme	1 slice	232	95	41
Skipper's				
Chicken basket				
5 strips and fries	1 basket	793	342	43
3 strips, 1 fish fillet and fries	1 basket	804	360	45
3 strips, orginal shrimp and fries	1 basket	800	351	44
Chicken sandwich	1 sandwich	606	288	48
Chicken strips	1 strip	82	36	44
Clam chowder	1 cup	100	32	32
Cod	1 piece	94	41	44
Cod, 3 pieces with fries	1 basket	665	288	43
Coleslaw	1/2 cup	289	243	84

FOOD		CALORIES		
	AMOUNT	TOTAL	FAT	%FAT
Fish fillet, 2.5 oz	1 fillet	175	90	51
Fish sandwich	1 sandwich	524	297	57
double	1 sandwich	698	657	94
French fries	1 serving	383	162	42
Jello	1/2 cup	55	0	0
Lite Catch Meals				
3 chicken strips and salad	1 basket	310	135	44
1 fish fillet, 2 chicken strips and salad	1 basket	403	189	47
2 fish fillets and salad	1 basket	413	207	50
Salad, shrimp and seafood	1 salad	175	45	26
Seafood basket				
clam strips and fries	1 basket	1003	630	63
original shrimp and fries	1 basket	723	324	45
Skipper's platter and fries	1 basket	1038	567	55
Seafood combo basket				
original shrimp, 1 fish fillet and fries	1 basket	728	333	46
oysters, 1 fish fillet and fries	1 basket	885	396	45
Taco Bell				
Burrito				
bean	1 burrito	357	92	26
beef	1 burrito	403	156	39
double beef supreme	1 burrito	457	196	43
supreme	1 burrito	413	158	38
Cinnamon Crispas	1 serving	259	138	53
Enchirito	1 serving	382	177	46
Fajita				
chicken	1 serving	226	92	41
steak	1 serving	233	98	42
Guacamole	1 serving	34	21	61

FOOD		CALORIES		
	AMOUNT	TOTAL	FAT	%FAT
Maximelt	1 serving	266	139	52
Mexican pizza	1 serving	575	331	58
Nachos	1 serving	346	167	48
Bellgrande	1 serving	649	318	49
Pico de Gallo	1 serving	8	?	25
Pintos and cheese	1 serving	190	78	41
Salsa	1 serving	18	8	44
Taco	1 taco	183	97	53
Bellgrande	1 taco	355	207	58
Light	1 taco	410	259	63
Taco, soft	1 taco	228	106	47
Supreme	1 taco	275	147	53
Taco salad with shell, with salsa	1 salad	941	552	59
without shell, with salsa	1 salad	520	283	54
Taco sauce, regular	1 packet	2	tr	tr
hot	1 packet	3	tr	tr
Tostada	1 serving	243	100	41
Wendy's				
Bacon Swiss burger	1 burger	710	396	56
Big Classic	1 burger	580	306	53
with cheese	1 burger	640	360	56
Breakfast sandwich	1 sandwich	370	171	46
Buttermilk biscuit	1 biscuit	320	153	48
Cheeseburger, plain, 1/4 pound	1 burger	410	198	48
single with everything	1 burger	490	252	51
small	1 burger	320	135	42
Chef salad	1 salad	180	81	45
Chicken fried steak	6 oz	580	369	64
Chicken nuggets	6 pieces	310	189	61
Chicken sandwich	1 sandwich	430	171	40

FOOD

CALORIES

	AMOUNT	TOTAL	FAT	%FAT
Chili	1 cup	230	81	35
Chocolate chip cookies	1 cookie	320	153	48
Danish				
apple	1 roll	360	126	35
cheese	1 roll	430	189	44
cinnamon raisin	1 roll	410	162	40
Fish fillet sandwich	1 sandwich	210	99	47
French fries, 3 oz	1 serving	300	135	45
French toast	2 slices	400	171	43
apple topping	1 packet	130	tr	tr
blueberry	1 packet	60	tr	tr
Frosty dairy dessert				
large	20 oz	666	210	32
medium	16 oz	533	168	32
small	12 oz	400	126	32
Garden salad	1 salad	120	45	44
Hamburger				
plain, 1/4 pound	1 burger	350	144	41
single with everything	1 burger	430	198	46
small	1 burger	260	81	31
Omelets				
cheese	1 omelet	290	189	65
cheese, mushroom	1 omelet	250	153	61
ham, cheese, green pepper, onion	1 omelet	280	171	61
mushroom, green pepper, onion	1 omelet	210	135	64
Philly Swiss burger	1 burger	510	216	42
Potato, baked, 9 oz				
plain	1 large	250	18	7
with bacon and cheese	1 large	570	270	47
with broccoli and cheese	1 large	500	225	45
with cheese	1 large	590	306	52
with chili and cheese	1 large	510	180	35
with sour cream and chives	1 large	460	216	47
Potatoes, breakfast, 3 oz	1 serving	360	198	55
Sausage gravy	6 oz	440	324	74
Sausage patty	1 1/2 oz	200	162	81

FOOD		CALORIES		
	AMOUNT	TOTAL	FAT	%FAT
Special sauce	1 Tbsp	40	27	68
Taco salad	1 salad	660	333	50

FATS AND OILS

Butter Buds, reconstituted	1 Tbsp	6	0	0
	1 oz	12	0	0
Butter				
regular	1 tsp	34	34	100
	1 pat	36	36	100
	1 Tbsp	102	102	100
	1 cup	1625	1625	100
whipped	1 tsp	23	23	100
	1 Tbsp	67	67	100
	1 cup	1081	1081	100
Lard	1 Tbsp	117	117	100
	1 cup	1849	1849	100
Margarine				
diet	1 tsp	17	17	100
	1 Tbsp	50	50	100
	1 cup	815	815	100
soft, tub, regular	1 tsp	34	34	100
	1 Tbsp	102	102	100
	1 cup	1634	1634	100
stick, regular	1 tsp	34	34	100
	1 pat	36	36	100
	1 Tbsp	102	102	100
	1 cup	1634	1634	100
whipped "lite"	1 tsp	23	23	100
	1 Tbsp	68	68	100
	1 cup	1087	1087	100

FOOD		CALORIES		
	AMOUNT	TOTAL	FAT	%FAT
Oil, salad or cooking, all types	1 tsp	40	40	100
	1 Tbsp	120	120	100
	1 cup	1927	1927	100
Shortening, vegetable, solid	1 Tbsp	111	111	100
	1 cup	1776	1776	100

FISH AND SHELLFISH

Abalone, raw	1 oz	30	2	6
Anchovies				
canned in oil	1 oz	60	25	42
pickled	1 oz	49	26	53
Bass, Sea, broiled	1 oz	35	6	17
Bluefish, broiled or baked	1 oz	44	13	30
Caviar, Sturgeon	1 Tbsp	42	22	52
Clam juice	1 cup	6	tr	tr
Clams				
breaded, fried ✔	1 oz	57	28	49
steamed or canned	1 oz	42	5	12
Cod, broiled or baked	1 oz	30	2	7
Crab, Alaska King, steamed	1 oz	27	4	15
Blue, canned	1 oz	28	3	11
Dungeness				
steamed	1 oz	26	5	19
flaked	1 cup	116	21	18
pieces	1 cup	144	26	18
White, canned	1 oz	29	6	21
	1 cup	135	26	19
Crab cocktail	2 oz	52	9	17
Crab Louis ✔	1 salad	642	495	77
Crab meat, imitation	1 oz	29	3	10

FOOD

CALORIES

	AMOUNT	TOTAL	FAT	%FAT
Fish Creole ✔	4 oz fish	351	108	31
Fish fillet, breaded, fried (Skipper's)	2.5 oz	175	90	51
Fish Florentine ✔	4 oz fish	240	108	45
Flounder				
broiled	1 oz	33	4	12
stuffed ✔	4 oz fish	311	153	49
Gefiltefish, sweet	1 oz	18	5	28
Grouper, broiled	1 oz	34	3	9
Haddock, broiled	1 oz	32	2	6
Halibut				
broiled	1 oz	40	7	18
smoked	1 oz	33	5	15
Herring, Atlantic, baked	1 oz	58	30	52
canned in tomato sauce	1 oz	50	27	54
kippered	1 oz	60	33	55
pickled	1 oz	78	54	69
Lobster				
grilled, with butter	5 oz	232	117	50
steamed	1 oz	28	2	7
Lox	1 oz	33	11	33
Lutefisk, raw	1 oz	30	3	10
Mackerel				
broiled	1 oz	75	46	61
canned	1 oz	51	26	51
Mussels, steamed	1 oz	49	12	24
Octopus, raw	1 oz	21	2	10
Oyster stew ✔	1 cup	233	138	59
Oysters Rockefeller ✔	6 oysters	200	99	50
Oysters				
breaded, fried, large, 1 oz	1 whole	56	32	57
Pacific, raw	1 oz	26	5	19
	1 cup	218	48	22
large	1 whole	52	11	21
medium	1 whole	38	8	21
small	1 whole	24	5	21
steamed	1 oz	39	13	33

FOOD

CALORIES

	AMOUNT	TOTAL	FAT	%FAT
Perch, broiled	1 oz	33	3	9
Pollack, Walleye, broiled	1 oz	32	3	9
Prawns, raw	1 oz	23	1	4
Red snapper, broiled	1 oz	36	4	11
Rockfish, broiled	1 oz	35	5	14
Salmon loaf, 2 x 2 x 3" slice ✔	1 slice	341	135	40
Salmon				
Atlantic, raw	1 oz	40	15	38
Chinook, smoked	1 oz	33	11	33
Coho/Silver, poached	1 oz	52	19	37
Humpback/Pink, canned	1 oz	39	15	38
Sockeye, broiled	1 oz	62	28	45
Sardines				
canned in oil, drained	1 oz	59	29	49
canned in tomato sauce	1 oz	50	31	62
Scallops				
breaded, fried ✔	1 oz	61	28	46
steamed	1 oz	32	3	9
Sea Bass, broiled	1 oz	35	6	17
Shark, raw	1 oz	37	12	32
Shad, baked	1 oz	57	29	51
Shrimp chow mein ✔	1 1/2 cups	455	153	34
Shrimp cocktail ✔	2 oz shrimp	106	9	8
Shrimp crepes (Mrs. Smith's)	2 crepes	305	144	47
Shrimp Newburg ✔	1 cup	572	387	68
Shrimp				
breaded, 1 shrimp = 1/2 oz	1 oz	69	31	45
canned	1 oz	28	3	11
steamed, 4 medium = 1 oz	1 oz	28	3	11
Sole, broiled	1 oz	23	2	9
Squid, steamed	1 oz	30	3	10
Stuffed flounder ✔	4 oz fish	311	153	49
Sturgeon				
smoked	1 oz	48	11	23
steamed	1 oz	39	14	36
Swordfish, broiled	1 oz	44	13	30

FOOD

CALORIES

	AMOUNT	TOTAL	FAT	%FAT
Trout Amandine ✔	4 oz fish	264	180	68
Trout, Rainbow, broiled	1 oz	43	11	26
Tuna				
Bluefin, broiled	1 oz	53	16	30
light, canned in oil	1 oz	56	21	38
canned in water	1 oz	37	1	3
white, canned in oil	1 oz	53	21	40
canned in water	1 oz	39	6	15
Whitefish, smoked	1 oz	31	2	6
Whiting, broiled	1 oz	33	4	12

FROZEN DINNERS AND ENTREES

	AMOUNT	TOTAL	FAT	%FAT
Beef Fajitas (Weight Watchers)	6 3/4 oz	260	54	21
Beef Pepper Steak (Tyson)	11 1/4 oz	330	99	30
Beef Stroganoff (Armour)	10 oz	320	108	34
Cheese Pizza (Banquet Kid Cuisine)	6.5 oz	240	36	15
Chicken a L' Orange (Lean Cuisine)	8 oz	260	54	21
Chicken Burrito (Weight Watchers)	7.62 oz	330	126	38
Chicken Cacciatori (Budget Gourmet)	11 oz	300	117	39
Chicken Chow Mein (Stouffer's)	8 oz	140	45	32
Chicken Fricassee (Armour)	11 3/4 oz	340	99	29
Chicken Kiev (Le Menu)	8 oz	530	351	66
Chicken 'n Dumplings (Banquet)	7 oz	280	126	45
Chicken Nuggets (Banquet Kid Cuisine)	6.25 oz	400	171	43
Chicken Nuggets (Swanson)				
3 oz = 5 nuggets	3 oz	250	144	58
Chicken Oriental dinner (Healthy Choice)	11 1/4 oz	220	18	8
Chicken Patties (Country Pride)	3 oz	232	135	58
Chicken Picatta (Tyson)	9 oz	240	90	38

FOOD

CALORIES

	AMOUNT	TOTAL	FAT	%FAT
Chicken Tamale Platter (Swanson)	9 3/4 oz	360	135	38
Chicken, Breast of, Marsala (Lean Cuisine)	8 1/8 oz	190	45	24
Egg Rolls				
chicken (La Choy)	3 rolls	69	26	38
restaurant style	3 oz	180	54	30
shrimp (La Choy)	3 rolls	62	21	34
Enchilada dinner (Swanson)				
beef	13 3/4 oz	480	198	41
chicken	9 oz	290	90	31
Enchiladas (El Charrito)				
beef	11 oz	560	279	50
cheese	11 oz	470	180	38
chicken	11 oz	440	117	27
Fish Fillets, battered (Van de Kamp's)				
1 fillet = 2 1/2 oz	2 1/2 oz	170	81	48
Fish 'n Chips (Swanson)				
1 fillet = 3 1/4 oz	3 1/4 oz	175	77	44
Fish 'n Chips dinner (Swanson)	10 oz	500	180	36
Fish Sticks, breaded (Van de Kamp's)	4 sticks	190	90	47
Fried Chicken, Original (Banquet)	6.4 oz	330	171	52
Hot 'n Spicy	6.4 oz	330	171	52
Fried Chicken dinner (Banquet)	10 oz	400	180	45
Fried Rice (Chung King)				
with chicken	8 oz	260	36	14
with pork	8 oz	270	54	20
Ham and Asparagus Au Gratin				
(Budget Gourmet Slim Selects)	9 oz	280	90	32
Lasagna with Meat Sauce (Stouffer's)	21 oz	720	234	33
	10 1/2 oz	360	117	33
Linguini with Scallops and Clams				
(Budget Gourmet Slim Selects)	9 1/2 oz	280	99	35
Macaroni and Cheeese dinner (Swanson)	12 1/4 oz	380	135	36
Macaroni and Cheese				
with Mini-Franks (Banquet Kid Cuisine)	9 oz	380	126	33
Mandarin Chicken (Budget Gourmet)	10 oz	290	54	19
Manicotti Milano (Stouffer's)	10 oz	360	180	50

FOOD

CALORIES

	AMOUNT	TOTAL	FAT	%FAT
Meat Loaf dinner (Swanson)	10 3/4 oz	430	198	46
Mexican Style Combination dinner				
(Swanson)	14 1/4 oz	520	216	42
My Meatballs and Shells (My Own Meals)	8 oz	210	81	39
Oriental Beef (Budget Gourmet Slim Selects)	10 oz	290	81	28
Oriental Beef with Vegetables and Rice				
(Lean Cuisine)	8 5/8 oz	250	63	25
Pasta Carbonara (Stouffer's)	7 3/4 oz	620	405	65
Pasta Primavera (Weight Watchers)	8 1/4 oz	290	117	40
Pepper Steak with Rice (Budget Gourmet)	10 oz	300	81	27
Pizza, 12" diameter				
Candian bacon, thin crust	1 pizza	1449	423	29
double topping no meat	1 pizza	2402	891	37
with meat	1 pizza	2483	1017	41
sausage, pepperoni or hamburger				
thin crust	1 pizza	1507	486	32
Pizza, 1/8 of 12" diameter				
Candian bacon, thin crust	1 slice	181	53	29
double topping no meat	1 slice	301	111	37
with meat	1 slice	310	127	41
sausage, pepperoni or hamburger				
thin crust	1 slice	188	61	32
Pot Pie (Swanson)				
beef	7 oz	380	180	47
chicken	7 oz	380	198	52
turkey	7 oz	380	198	52
Salisibury Steak dinner (Swanson)	10 3/4 oz	430	180	42
(Swanson Hungry Man)	16 1/2 oz	610	315	52
Shrimp Fried Rice, frozen (Green Giant)	10 oz	300	45	15
Sirlion Enchilada Ranchero				
(Budget Gourmet Slim Select)	9 oz	290	135	47
Sirlion Tips dinner (Healthy Choice)	11 3/4 oz	290	54	19
Sirlion Tips with Burgundy Sauce dinner				
(Budget Gourmet)	11 oz	310	99	32
Sole au Gratin dinner (Healthy Choice)	11 1/2 oz	280	45	6
Spaghetti with Meatballs (Swanson)	12 1/2 oz	370	144	39

FOOD

CALORIES

	AMOUNT	TOTAL	FAT	%FAT
Spaghetti with Meat Sauce (Stouffer's)	12 7/8 oz	370	99	27
Swedish Meatballs with Noodles (Budget Gourmet)	10 oz	600	351	59
Sweet and Sour Chicken dinner (Healthy Choice)	11 1/2 oz	280	18	6
Sweet 'n Sour Chicken with Rice (Budget Gourmet)	10 oz	350	63	18
Swiss Steak dinner (Swanson)	10 oz	350	99	28
Sylvester Fish Sticks (Tyson Looney Tunes Meals)	7.3 oz	270	99	37
Teriyaki Chicken (Budget Gourmet)	12 oz	360	108	30
Tortellini with Cheese Sauce (Budget Gourmet)	5 1/2 oz	180	54	30
Tortellini,Cheese, Alfredo (Stouffer's)	8 7/8 oz	600	360	60
Tuna Noodle Casserole (Swanson)	9 oz	260	99	38
Turkey Dijon (Lean Cuisine)	9 1/2 oz	270	90	33
Turkey Dinner (Swanson)	9 oz	280	99	35
Turkey Tetrazini (Stouffer's)	10 oz	380	180	47
Veal Parmigiana dinner (Swanson)	12 1/4 oz	450	189	42
Vegetable Chow Mein (La Choy)	1 cup	69	3	4
Zucchini Lasagna (Lean Cuisine)	11 oz	260	63	24

FRUIT JUICES

	AMOUNT	TOTAL	FAT	%FAT
Apple juice canned or frozen, reconstituted, unsweetened	8 oz	120	tr	tr
frozen, concentrate	6 oz	270	tr	tr
Apricot nectar, canned	8 oz	145	tr	tr
Cran-raspberry juice, bottled (Ocean Spray)	8 oz	144	tr	tr
Cranapple juice, bottled (Ocean Spray)	8 oz	168	tr	tr

FOOD

CALORIES

	AMOUNT	TOTAL	FAT	%FAT
Cranberry apple juice, bottled	8 oz	172	2	1
Cranberry juice, bottled, sweetened	8 oz	165	1	1
low calorie, bottled	8 oz	48	4	8
Fruit Punch, (Hawaiian Punch)	8 oz	120	tr	tr
"lite" (Hawaiian Punch)	8 oz	107	tr	tr
Grape drink, canned	8 oz	135	tr	tr
Grape juice				
canned, bottled or				
frozen reconstituted	8 oz	165	tr	tr
frozen, concentrate, sweetened	6 oz	395	tr	tr
Grapefruit juice				
canned, sweetened	8 oz	135	tr	tr
fresh or frozen,				
reconstituted, unsweetened	8 oz	100	tr	tr
frozen, concentrate	6 oz	300	8	3
Lemon juice, fresh, canned or				
bottled, unsweetened	1 Tbsp	3	tr	tr
	8 oz	55	tr	tr
Lemonade, frozen, concentrate	6 oz	425	tr	tr
reconstituted	8 oz	105	tr	tr
Lime juice, fresh or canned, unsweetened	1 Tbsp	4	tr	tr
	8 oz	65	tr	tr
Limeade, frozen, concentrate	6 oz	410	tr	tr
reconstituted	8 oz	100	tr	tr
Orange juice				
canned or frozen,				
reconstituted, unsweetened	8 oz	120	tr	tr
dehydrated crystals, reconstituted	8 oz	115	tr	tr
frozen, concentrate	6 oz	360	tr	tr
Orange/grapefruit juice				
frozen, concentrate	6 oz	330	8	2
reconstituted	8 oz	110	tr	tr
Pineapple juice				
canned, unsweetened	8 oz	138	tr	tr
frozen, concentrate	6 oz	387	3	1
frozen, reconstituted	8 oz	130	1	1

FOOD		CALORIES		
	AMOUNT	TOTAL	FAT	%FAT
Prune juice, canned or bottled	8 oz	195	tr	tr
Tangerine juice, canned, unsweetened	8 oz	125	tr	tr

FRUITS

FOOD	AMOUNT	TOTAL	FAT	%FAT
Apple, fresh, 3" diameter	1 apple	96	8	8
Apples, dried	1 oz	83	8	10
1.4 oz = 1/2 cup	1/2 cup	117	6	5
Applesauce, canned				
sweetened	1/2 cup	115	tr	tr
unsweetened	1/2 cup	50	tr	tr
Apricots dried, 4 halves	1 oz	74	1	1
2.7 oz = 1/2 cup	1/2 cup	200	3	2
Apricots				
canned				
heavy syrup	1/2 cup	110	tr	tr
juice pack	1/2 cup	54	2	4
water pack	1/2 cup	38	1	3
fresh, whole	3 apricots	55	2	4
Avocado				
cubed	1/2 cup	125	110	88
mashed	1/2 cup	276	243	88
whole, peeled, 4" diameter	1 average	378	333	88
Banana chips, dehydrated	1 oz	103	10	10
Banana flakes	1 Tbsp	20	tr	tr
Banana, medium, 7"	1 banana	100	2	2
Blackberries, fresh	1/2 cup	43	4	9
Blueberries, fresh	1/2 cup	45	4	9
Boysenberries, fresh, canned or				
frozen, unsweetened	1/2 cup	44	1	2

FOOD

CALORIES

	AMOUNT	TOTAL	FAT	%FAT
Cantaloupe, fresh, 5" diameter	1/2 melon	82	3	4
cubed	1/2 cup	24	2	8
Casaba melon, fresh, 6 1/2" diameter,				
2" wedge	1 wedge	38	tr	tr
Cherimoya	1 average	515	20	4
Cherries				
fresh	10 cherries	45	tr	tr
Maraschino, large	1 cherry	10	0	0
canned				
sour/red, water pack	1/2 cup	53	tr	tr
in heavy syrup	1/2 cup	116	tr	tr
sweet, water pack	1/2 cup	43	2	5
juice pack	1/2 cup	68	tr	tr
Crab apples, fresh, sliced	1/2 cup	68	3	4
Cranberries, fresh, whole	1/2 cup	22	3	14
Cranberry sauce, canned, sweetened	1/4 cup	102	2	2
Currants, dried	1/4 cup	100	4	4
Dates				
chopped	1/2 cup	245	4	2
whole, without pits	1 date	22	tr	tr
Elderberries, fresh	1/2 cup	72	5	7
Figs, canned, whole				
in heavy syrup	1/2 cup	109	3	3
water pack	1/2 cup	60	2	3
Figs, fresh				
1 1/2" diameter	1 fig	32	1	3
2 1/4" diameter	1 fig	40	2	5
Fresh fruit cup	1 cup	104	tr	tr
Fruit cocktail, canned				
in heavy syrup	1/2 cup	76	1	1
juice pack	1/2 cup	50	1	2
water pack	1/2 cup	37	1	3
Gooseberries, fresh	1/2 cup	30	1	3
Grapefruit, canned				
sweetened	1/2 cup	70	1	1
unsweetened	1/2 cup	30	1	3

FOOD | CALORIES

	AMOUNT	TOTAL	FAT	%FAT
Grapefruit, fresh				
pink, 3 3/4" diameter	1/2 fruit	50	tr	tr
white, 3 3/4" diameter	1/2 fruit	45	tr	tr
Grapes, fresh, all varieties	10 grapes	40	tr	tr
Guava, fresh, medium	1 guava	62	5	8
Honeydew, fresh				
6 1/2" diameter, 2" wedge	1 wedge	50	4	8
cubed	1/2 cup	28	2	7
Kiwi, fresh, medium	1 kiwi	50	tr	tr
Kumquat, fresh, medium	1 kumquat	12	tr	tr
Lemon, fresh	1 lemon	20	tr	tr
Lime, fresh	1 lime	28	2	7
Loganberries, fresh	1/2 cup	45	4	9
Loquats, fresh	1 whole	6	tr	tr
Mandarin oranges, fresh, 2 3/8" diameter	1 average	37	tr	tr
canned, unsweetened	1/2 cup	31	4	13
Mango, fresh, medium	1 mango	152	7	5
Melon balls, cantaloupe or honeydew,				
frozen	1/2 cup	72	2	3
Mixed fruit, dried	1 oz	73	1	1
Muskmelon, fresh, 5" diameter	1/2 melon	82	3	4
Nectarine, fresh, 2 1/2" diameter	1 fruit	88	tr	tr
Orange				
fresh, 3" diameter	1 orange	73	tr	tr
sections	1/2 cup	45	tr	tr
Papaya, fresh				
1/2" cubes	1/2 cup	28	tr	tr
3 1/2" diameter	1 papaya	119	2	2
Peaches				
canned				
in heavy syrup	2 halves	78	1	1
sliced	1/2 cup	78	1	1
juice pack	2 halves	45	1	2
water pack	2 halves	31	1	3
sliced	1/2 cup	31	1	3
dried	1/2 cup	210	4	2

FOOD

CALORIES

	AMOUNT	TOTAL	FAT	%FAT
Peaches (continued)				
fresh, 2 1/2" diameter	1 peach	40	tr	tr
sliced	1/2 cup	32	1	3
frozen, sliced, sweetened	1/2 cup	110	tr	tr
Pears				
canned, in heavy syrup	2 halves	76	2	3
water pack	2 halves	58	2	3
fresh, D'Anjou, 3" diameter	1 pear	120	8	7
Persimmon, fresh	1 fruit	103	2	2
Pineapple, canned				
chunks, juice pack	1/2 cup	40	tr	tr
crushed, in syrup	1/2 cup	95	tr	tr
slices, in heavy syrup	1 slice	74	1	1
tidbits, water pack	1/2 cup	48	tr	tr
Pineapple, dried	1 oz	74	3	4
Pineapple fresh, diced	1/2 cup	40	tr	tr
Plantain	1 plantain	119	4	3
Plums				
canned, in heavy syrup	3 plums	83	1	1
water pack	3 plums	44	1	2
fresh, 1 1/2" diameter	1 plum	20	tr	tr
2 1/8" diameter	1 plum	30	tr	tr
Pomegranate, pulp only, 2 3/8 x 3/8"	1 fruit	97	4	4
Prunes, dried				
cooked, unsweetened	1/2 cup	128	4	3
large	1 prune	25	0	0
Quince	1 average	53	1	2
Raisins, seedless	1 Tbsp	29	tr	tr
1/2 oz packet	1 packet	40	tr	tr
2.6 oz = 1/2 cup	1/2 cup	210	tr	tr
Rasberries, black,				
fresh or canned, unsweetened	1/2 cup	59	9	15
Raspberries, red				
fresh or canned, unsweetened	1/2 cup	43	1	2
frozen, sweetened	1/2 cup	123	2	2

FOOD

CALORIES

	AMOUNT	TOTAL	FAT	%FAT
Rhubarb, cooked				
unsweetened	1/2 cup	32	tr	tr
with 3 Tbsp sugar	1/2 cup	188	tr	tr
Rhubarb, raw, cubed	1 cup	16	tr	tr
Sapodilla	1 average	140	18	13
Starfruit, 4" diameter	1 average	42	3	7
Strawberries				
fresh, large	10 berries	37	5	14
frozen, sliced, sweetened	1/2 cup	140	2	1
whole, sweetened	1/2 cup	112	2	2
Tangerine, fresh, large	1 tangerine	46	2	4
Tangelo, fresh, medium	1 tangelo	39	1	3
Watermelon, fresh				
4 x 8" wedge	1 wedge	110	1	1
diced	1/2 cup	21	1	5

GRAINS AND GRAIN PRODUCTS

	AMOUNT	TOTAL	FAT	%FAT
Arrowroot	1 Tbsp	30	0	0
Barley, pearled, pot or Scotch				
cooked	1 cup	199	5	3
dry	1 cup	698	2	tr
Bean threads, cooked	1 cup	98	tr	tr
Bowties, pasta				
cooked	1 cup	100	9	9
dry	1 cup	200	18	9
Bran, oat	1 Tbsp	21	3	14
	1 cup	330	54	16
Bran, wheat, unprocessed or miller's	1 cup	111	22	20
	1 Tbsp	7	tr	tr

FOOD	CALORIES		
	AMOUNT	TOTAL	FAT	%FAT

FOOD	AMOUNT	TOTAL	FAT	%FAT
Bulgur, cooked	1 cup	226	9	4
dry	1 cup	600	23	4
Chinese fried rice ✔	1 cup	312	166	53
Cornmeal, yellow or white				
cooked	1 cup	120	5	4
dry	1 cup	530	16	3
Cornstarch	1 Tbsp	29	0	0
Couscous, cooked	1 cup	160	0	0
Curried rice ✔	1/2 cup	233	54	23
Farina, quick cook or regular, cooked	1 cup	105	2	2
Fettuccini, noodles				
cooked	1 cup	150	9	6
dry	1 cup	200	9	5
Fettuccini, spinach, cooked	1 cup	150	9	6
dry	1 cup	200	9	5
Flour				
all-purpose, white	1 Tbsp	29	1	3
	1 cup	400	10	3
barley	1 Tbsp	28	1	4
	1 cup	401	17	4
buckwheat, light or dark	1 Tbsp	22	1	5
	1 cup	347	11	3
gluten	1 Tbsp	33	2	6
	1 cup	529	24	5
potato	1 Tbsp	22	tr	0
	1 cup	351	7	2
rice	1 Tbsp	30	tr	tr
	1 cup	479	4	1
rye, dark	1 Tbsp	27	2	7
	1 cup	419	26	6
rye, light	1 Tbsp	20	1	5
	1 cup	314	8	3
soybean, low-fat	1 Tbsp	19	3	16
	1 cup	304	48	16
whole wheat	1 Tbsp	29	1	3
	1 cup	400	22	6

FOOD

CALORIES

	AMOUNT	TOTAL	FAT	%FAT
Gnocchi, cheese, baked ✔	1 cup	449	261	58
Grits, cooked	1 cup	125	tr	tr
Lasagna noodles, cut				
cooked	1 cup	200	12	6
dry	1 cup	225	13	6
long, dry, 3 noodles = 2 oz	2 oz	210	9	4
Lefse, 10" diameter ✔	1 lefse	79	15	19
Macaroni, cooked				
firm	1 cup	207	6	3
tender	1 cup	151	5	3
Macaroni, dry	1 cup	405	12	3
Macaroni, spinach				
cooked	1 cup	155	5	3
dry	1 cup	524	15	3
Manicotti, large noodle, dry	2 pieces	102	9	9
Matzo ball, 2" diameter	1 ball	123	74	60
Millet				
cooked	1 cup	165	13	8
dry	1 cup	660	53	8
Noodles, chow mein, hard, canned	1 cup	220	108	49
Noodles, plain				
cooked	1 cup	146	4	3
dry	1 cup	248	7	3
Noodles, egg				
cooked	1 cup	200	21	11
dry	1 cup	283	30	11
Noodles, spinach, cooked	1 cup	200	22	11
Oats, rolled				
cooked	1 cup	148	25	17
dry	1 cup	333	57	17
Orzo				
cooked	1 cup	210	9	4
dry	1 cup	630	27	4
Polenta ✔	1/3 cup	72	9	13
Popcorn				
air popped, unbuttered	1 cup	25	2	8

FOOD		CALORIES		
	AMOUNT	TOTAL	FAT	%FAT
Popcorn (continued)				
microwave, pouch type	1 cup	35	18	51
caramel	1 cup	96	50	52
cheddar cheese	1 cup	50	30	60
light	1 cup	17	3	18
oil popped, buttered with 2 tsp	1 cup	108	86	80
unbuttered	1 cup	40	18	45
unpopped	1 cup	742	84	11
Pretzels				
Dutch, 28 per lb	1 large	58	2	3
three ring, 148 per lb	1 piece	12	1	8
very thin sticks, 1600 per lb	1 piece	10	tr	tr
Rice noodles, cooked	1 cup	241	36	15
Rice pilaf ✔	1 cup	168	52	31
Rice, brown, instant, cooked	1 cup	240	18	8
Rice, brown, long-grain				
cooked	1 cup	232	14	6
dry	1 cup	666	39	6
Rice, brown, short-grain				
cooked	1 cup	240	11	5
dry	1 cup	720	33	5
Rice, brown, whole grain, fast cooking,				
cooked	1 cup	180	18	10
Rice, long grain and wild blend	1 cup	194	2	1
Rice, white, converted, cooked	1 cup	182	2	1
Rice, white, long-grain,				
cooked	1 cup	223	2	1
dry	1 cup	672	6	1
quick, cooked	1 cup	158	2	1
Rice, white, short-grain				
cooked	1 cup	275	2	1
dry	1 cup	726	7	1
Rice, wild				
cooked	1 cup	141	3	2
dry	1 cup	396	7	2
Rice, with red wheat, barley, cooked (Hain)	1 cup	180	18	10

FOOD		CALORIES		
	AMOUNT	TOTAL	FAT	%FAT
Rice-A-Roni				
beef	1/2 cup	110	9	8
chicken	1/2 cup	140	9	6
Spanish	1/2 cup	150	36	24
Rigatoni				
cooked	1 cup	100	6	6
dry	1 cup	200	12	6
Rotini, spirals				
cooked	1 cup	100	9	9
dry	1 cup	200	18	9
Shells, pasta				
cooked	1 cup	100	9	9
dry	1 cup	200	18	9
Spaghetti with meatballs ✔	1 cup	332	105	32
Spaghetti, pasta, cooked				
firm	1 cup	192	6	3
tender	1 cup	155	5	3
Spaghetti, dry	1 lb	1674	49	3
Spaghetti, spinach, cooked	1 cup	192	6	3
Spaghetti whole wheat, cooked				
firm	1 cup	183	13	7
tender	1 cup	152	11	7
Spaghetti, whole wheat, dry	1 lb	1600	117	7
Spanish rice ✔	1/2 cup	217	81	37
Taco salad shell, 2.5 oz	1 shell	421	269	64
Tapioca, dry	1 cup	535	3	1
	1 Tbsp	30	tr	tr
Tortellini, cooked				
cheese	1 cup	754	108	14
meat	1 cup	754	108	14
Tortilla, soft				
6" diameter				
corn	1 tortilla	63	5	8
flour	1 tortilla	95	18	19
whole wheat	1 tortilla	97	16	16
8" diameter, flour	1 tortilla	127	24	19

FOOD

CALORIES

	AMOUNT	TOTAL	FAT	%FAT
Vermicelli, coil				
cooked	1 cup	150	9	6
dry	1 cup	200	9	5
Wheat berries				
cooked	1 cup	221	16	7
dry	1 cup	578	42	7
Wheat bran, unprocessed or miller's	1 cup	121	23	19
	1 Tbsp	8	tr	tr
Wheat germ	1 Tbsp	23	6	26
2 oz = 1 cup	1 cup	368	101	27
Wheat, cracked				
cooked	1 cup	227	8	4
dry	1 cup	509	30	6
Wheat, rolled				
cooked	1 cup	180	8	4
dry	1 cup	405	18	4
Wheat, whole grain, cooked	1 cup	243	8	3
Whole wheat noodles, homemade ✔	1/2 cup	88	9	10
Wild rice				
cooked	1 cup	141	3	2
dry	1 cup	396	7	2

ICE CREAM AND FROZEN DESSERTS

Baked Alaska, 1/8 of 9 x 9 x 2" ✔	1 serving	557	21	4
Banana split (Dairy Queen)	1 serving	540	99	18
Buster bar (Dairy Queen)	1 serving	460	261	57

FOOD		CALORIES		
	AMOUNT	TOTAL	FAT	%FAT
Chocolate Mint Treat				
(Weight Watchers), 1 = 2.7 oz	1 serving	100	9	9
Cookies 'n Cream sandwich (Oreo)	1 bar	240	99	41
Creamsicle (Sealtest)	1 average	103	28	27
Dove Bar, 3.8 oz	1 bar	306	135	44
Light	1 bar	230	99	43
Drumstick, ice cream cone	1 average	186	89	48
Eskimo Pie, 3 oz	1 bar	180	108	60
Light, 2.5 oz	1 bar	140	81	57
Sugar free, 2.5 oz	1 bar	140	108	77
Frosty, dairy dessert, small (Wendy's)	12 oz	400	126	32
Frozen dessert, all flavors,				
7 x 3 1/2 x 1/2" (Weight Watchers)	1 slice	100	36	36
Fruit and Cream Bar (Chiquita)	1 bar	80	9	11
Fruit and Juice Bar, 2.5 oz (Dole)	1 bar	70	tr	tr
Fresh Lites, 1.65 oz	1 bar	25	tr	tr
Fruit and Yogurt Bar (Dole)	1 bar	70	tr	tr
Fudgsicle, 1.75 oz	1 bar	70	9	13
sugar free, 1.25 oz	1 bar	35	9	26
Gise, frozen dessert	1 cup	76	tr	tr
Ice cream				
(Baskin Robbins)	1 cup	470	236	50
sugar free	1 cup	200	36	18
brick, any flavor	1 cup	295	144	49
bulk (Breyers)	1 cup	300	144	48
(Haagen Dazs)	1 cup	546	306	56
Ice cream cone	1 cup	295	144	49
plain, without ice cream	1 cone	18	2	11
sugar, without ice cream	1 cone	49	39	80
waffle, without ice cream	1 average	118	25	21
Ice cream float (Dairy Queen)	1 serving	410	63	15
Ice cream sandwich, 2.5 oz	1 bar	162	45	28
Ice milk				
brick, 4.4 oz	1 cup	185	54	29
Dreyer's Grand Light	1 cup	240	90	38
soft serve, 5.8 oz	1 cup	225	45	20

FOOD | CALORIES

	AMOUNT	TOTAL	FAT	%FAT
Milkshake				
chocolate (Burger King)	1 shake	320	108	34
chocolate (Hardee's)	1 shake	460	72	16
chocolate (McDonald's)	1 shake	390	95	24
strawberry (McDonald's)	1 shake	380	91	24
vanilla (Burger King)	1 shake	321	90	28
vanilla (McDonald's)	1 shake	350	92	26
Mocha Mix, non-dairy dessert				
vanilla or strawberry	1 cup	280	126	45
chocolate, mocha or almond	1 cup	300	162	54
Popsicle				
(Jell-O)	1 average	30	tr	tr
(Crystal Light)	1 average	13	tr	tr
Pudding Pops (Jell O)	1 average	75	18	24
Sherbet, all varieties	1 cup	270	36	13
Simple Pleasures, frozen dessert				
chocolate	1 cup	280	tr	tr
strawberry	1 cup	240	tr	tr
Strawberry Shortcake bar, 3 oz				
(Good Humor)	1 bar	186	108	58
Soft serve with cone (Dairy Queen)	1 small	140	36	26
	1 large	340	90	26
dipped (Dairy Queen)	1 small	190	80	42
	1 large	510	216	42
Sorbet (Dole)	1 cup	240	tr	tr
Sundae, soft serve (McDonald's)				
hot caramel	1 sundae	340	82	24
hot fudge	1 sundae	310	85	27
strawberry	1 sundae	280	66	23
Tofutti, frozen dessert				
Lite, Lite	1 cup	180	tr	tr
vanilla, regular	1 cup	400	198	50
Vitari, frozen fruit treat	1 cup	160	tr	tr
Yogurt, frozen, low-fat				
(Dannon)	1 cup	240	26	11
(Honey Hill Farms)	1 cup	210	56	27

FOOD		CALORIES		
	AMOUNT	TOTAL	FAT	%FAT
Yogurt, frozen, low-fat (continued)				
(I Can't Believe It's Yogurt)	1 cup	288	65	23
(TCBY)	1 cup	240	72	30
(Tuscan Farms)	1 cup	220	18	8
Gourmet (Yo Cream)	1 cup	240	72	30
Yogurt, frozen, non-fat				
(I Can't Believe It's Yogurt)	1 cup	224	18	8
(TCBY)	1 cup	200	18	9
Lite (Yo Cream)	1 cup	200	34	17
Yogurt, frozen, non-fat, sugar free				
(Honey Hill Farms)	1 cup	80	tr	tr

JAMS AND JELLIES

Apple butter	1 Tbsp	33	1	3
Jam and jelly, all varieties				
regular	1 tsp	18	tr	tr
	1 Tbsp	55	tr	tr
1/2 oz packet	1 packet	40	tr	tr
low sugar	1 Tbsp	24	tr	tr
	1 tsp	8	tr	tr
Pectin				
Certo, liquid	1/2 cup	12	0	0
Sure-Jell, dry	1 oz	76	0	0

FOOD

CALORIES

	AMOUNT	TOTAL	FAT	%FAT

LEGUMES

Food	AMOUNT	TOTAL	FAT	%FAT
Baked beans, canned				
with pork, tomato sauce	1/2 cup	156	30	19
with sweet sauce	1/2 cup	191	54	28
vegetarian, without pork	1/2 cup	153	6	4
Bean threads, cooked	1 cup	98	tr	tr
Beans, refried, plain or spicy	1 cup	248	16	6
Black beans				
cooked	1 cup	280	12	4
dry	1 cup	678	28	4
Blackeyed peas, cowpeas				
cooked	1 cup	178	12	7
raw	1 cup	184	10	5
Chickpeas, garbanzo or ceci beans				
cooked	1 cup	338	41	12
dry	1 cup	720	86	12
Chili con carne with beans, canned (Stokley)	1 cup	390	234	60
Cowpeas or blackeyed peas				
cooked	1 cup	178	12	7
raw	1 cup	184	10	5
Fava or broad beans, dry	1 lb	1533	69	5
Garbanzo, chickpeas, ceci beans				
cooked	1 cup	338	41	12
dry	1 cup	720	86	12

FOOD

CALORIES

	AMOUNT	TOTAL	FAT	%FAT
Great Northern beans, white				
cooked	1 cup	212	10	5
dry	1 cup	612	26	4
Hummus ✔	1/4 cup	105	47	45
Kidney beans				
canned	1 cup	135	6	4
cooked	1 cup	218	8	4
dry	1 cup	635	25	4
Lentils				
cooked	1 cup	210	tr	tr
dry	1 cup	680	10	1
Lima beans, large				
cooked	1 cup	276	11	4
dry	1 cup	690	29	4
Lima beans, small				
cooked	1 cup	262	10	4
dry	1 cup	656	27	4
Mung bean sprouts, raw	1 cup	37	2	5
Mung beans				
cooked	1 cup	355	12	3
dry	1 cup	714	24	3
Navy or pea beans				
cooked	1 cup	224	10	4
dry	1 cup	697	30	4
Peas, split				
cooked	1 cup	230	5	2
dry	1 cup	696	18	3
Peas, whole				
cooked	1 cup	338	11	3
dry	1 cup	680	23	3
Pinto or calico beans				
cooked	1 cup	288	9	3
dry	1 cup	663	20	3
Pork and beans	1 cup	237	18	8
Refried beans, plain or spicy	1 cup	248	16	6
vegetarian	1 cup	225	34	15

FOOD		CALORIES		
	AMOUNT	TOTAL	FAT	%FAT
Soybeans				
sprouted seeds, cooked or raw	1 cup	48	16	33
whole				
cooked	1 cup	234	93	40
dry	1 cup	846	335	40
Tofu, soybean curd	1/2 cup	81	43	53
	1 lb	331	174	53
2 1/2 x 2 3/4 x 1"	1 piece	86	45	52
TVP, textured vegetable protein, dehydrated	1 oz	101	2	2

Meats and Meat Products

FOOD	AMOUNT	TOTAL	FAT	%FAT
Bac-O-Bits (General Mills)	1 Tbsp	38	14	37
Bacon				
broiled or fried, crisp	2 slices	85	72	85
Canadian	1 oz	61	37	61
Imitation Crubles (R.T. French)	1 tsp	6	tr	tr
Beef (Land O'Frost)	1 oz	40	18	45
Beef jerky	1 oz	108	43	40
Beef Kebabs ✔	1 kebab	358	207	58
Beef teriyaki ✔	4 oz beef	429	315	73
Beef tongue, simmered	1 oz	80	53	66
Beef				
brisket, braised	1 oz	68	33	49
chuck, arm pot roast, braised	1 oz	65	25	38
dried	1 oz	47	10	21

FOOD   CALORIES

	AMOUNT	TOTAL	FAT	%FAT
Beef (continued)				
ground				
extra lean, 15% fat				
1 lb raw = 12 oz cooked	12 oz	804	444	55
baked	1 oz	67	36	54
broiled	1 oz	68	37	54
pan-fried	1 oz	67	37	55
lean, 20% fat				
1 lb raw = 11 1/2 oz cooked	11 1/2 oz	886	541	61
baked	1 oz	75	45	60
broiled	1 oz	76	46	60
pan-fried	1 oz	77	47	61
regular, 27% fat				
1 lb raw = 11 oz cooked	11 oz	957	649	68
baked	1 oz	82	54	66
broiled	1 oz	83	54	65
pan-fried	1 oz	87	59	68
heart, simmered	1 oz	49	14	29
eye of round, roasted	1 oz	52	17	33
liver, fried	1 oz	65	27	42
rib				
large end, roasted	1 oz	69	36	52
small end, roasted	1 oz	62	29	47
short ribs, braised	1 oz	84	46	55
top round, broiled	1 oz	54	16	30
Bockwurst	1 oz	74	59	80
Bologna	1 oz	88	73	83
Braunschweiger	1 oz	102	82	80
Brotwurst	1 oz	90	72	80
Calf liver				
fried	1 oz	75	34	45
raw	1 oz	40	12	30
Chicken fried round steak ✔	4 oz	363	225	62
Chorizo, pork and beef	2 oz link	265	207	78
Corn dog	1 serving	345	202	59
Corned beef hash	1 cup	398	224	56

FOOD | CALORIES

	AMOUNT	TOTAL	FAT	%FAT
Corned beef, boneless				
canned	1 oz	61	31	51
cooked	1 oz	71	48	68
Deviled ham, canned	1 Tbsp	45	36	80
Gravy, beef				
brown, dry, mix, reconstituted	1/4 cup	2	1	50
canned	1/4 cup	31	13	42
with fat drippings ✔	1/4 cup	164	126	77
Gravy, sausage (Wendy's)	6 oz	440	324	74
Ham				
canned				
lean, 4% fat	1 oz	39	12	31
regular, 13% fat	1 oz	64	39	61
luncheon				
extra lean, 5% fat	1 oz	37	9	24
regular, 11% fat	1 oz	52	27	52
picnic, roasted	1 oz	65	32	49
diced, 1 cup = 4.5 oz	1 cup	293	144	49
whole, roasted	1 oz	62	28	45
Ham salad spread	1 oz	61	40	66
Hot dog				
5" x 3/4", 10 per lb	1.6 oz	139	109	78
5" x 7/8", 8 per lb	2 oz	176	138	78
Jerky, beef	1 oz	108	43	40
Kielbasa	1 oz	88	69	79
Knockwurst	1 oz	87	71	82
Lamb chop with bone, broiled	1.7 oz	92	36	39
Lamb shoulder, whole, braised	1 oz	80	41	51
Leg of lamb, whole, roasted	1 oz	54	20	37
Liver sausage	1 oz	97	81	84
Liver				
beef, fried	1 oz	65	27	42
calf, fried	1 oz	75	34	45
raw	1 oz	40	12	30
Liverwurst spread	1 oz	91	69	76
Meat, canned, potted	1 Tbsp	30	18	60

FOOD

CALORIES

FOOD	AMOUNT	TOTAL	FAT	%FAT
Pastrami	1 oz	106	78	74
Pepperoni	1 oz	141	112	79
Polish sausage				
10" x 1 1/4"	8 oz	690	516	75
5 3/8" x 1"	2.7 oz	231	172	74
Pork chop				
sirloin, broiled	1 oz	69	34	49
center loin, broiled	1 oz	65	27	42
top loin, broiled	1 oz	73	38	52
Pork feet, simmered	1 oz	55	31	56
Pork links, cooked	1 oz	110	81	74
Pork sausage, cooked				
(Brown and Serve)	1 oz	118	95	81
regular	1/2 cup	280	211	75
Pork shoulder, whole, roasted	1 oz	69	38	55
Pork, shoulder, Boston blade, roasted	1 oz	73	43	59
Pot roast, beef, cooked	1 oz	65	25	38
Rabbit, domestic, stewed	1 oz	61	27	44
Salami	1 oz	111	84	76
Light and Lean (Hormel)	3/4 oz	40	27	68
Genoa	1 oz	110	90	82
hard	1 oz	115	86	75
Salt pork, raw	1 oz	212	205	97
Sausage				
(Brown and Serve), browned	1 link	70	54	77
bulk or links, cooked	1 oz	110	81	74
cholesterol free	1 oz	80	45	56
Polish, 10" x 1 1/4"	8 oz	690	516	75
5 3/8" x 1"	2.7 oz	231	172	74
pork, cooked	1/2 cup	280	211	75
	1 oz	105	79	75
summer, beef stick (Hickory Farms)	1 oz	100	72	72
Spam (Hormel)	1 oz	87	67	77
Spareribs, pork, braised	1 oz	113	77	68
Sportsman stick (Hickory Farms)	1 oz	138	90	65

FOOD | CALORIES

	AMOUNT	TOTAL	FAT	%FAT
Steak, beef				
cubed, cooked	1 oz	75	40	53
flank, broiled	1 oz	69	38	55
porterhouse. broiled	1 oz	62	28	45
sirlon, broiled	1 oz	58	18	31
T-bone, broiled	1 oz	61	26	43
top loin, broiled	1 oz	57	23	40
top round, broiled	1 oz	54	16	30
Stuffed pork chops ✔	1 chop	802	585	73
Summer sausage, beef stick	1 oz	100	72	72
Swiss steak, 3 x 3 x 1/2" ✔	1 piece	214	81	38
Veal				
cutlets, pan fried	1 oz	58	16	28
loln, boneless, braised	1 oz	64	23	36
shoulder, braised	1 oz	56	16	29
Venison				
cooked	1 oz	57	16	28
raw	1 oz	35	9	26

MEXICAN FOODS

	AMOUNT	TOTAL	FAT	%FAT
Bean dip, canned (Frito Lay)	1/4 cup	66	25	38
Beans, refried, plain or spicy	1 cup	248	16	6
vegetarian	1 cup	225	34	15
Burrito, Chicken, frozen (Weight Watchers)	7.62 oz	330	126	38
Burrito Supreme (Taco Bell)	1 burrito	413	158	38
Burrito				
bean (Taco Bell)	1 burrito	357	92	26
bean and cheese, 5 oz	1 burrito	339	99	29
beef (Taco Bell)	1 burrito	403	156	93

FOOD

CALORIES

	AMOUNT	TOTAL	FAT	%FAT
Burrito (continued)				
beef and bean, 5 oz	1 burrito	366	135	37
green chili, 5 oz	1 burrito	353	117	33
red hot beef, 5 oz	1 burrito	319	109	34
Chili relleno, with cheese, fried ✔	1 serving	146	95	65
Chilies, green	1 Tbsp	4	0	0
Corn chips				
10 chips = 1 oz (Tostitos)	1 oz	150	72	48
15 chips = 1 oz (Doritos)	1 oz	140	56	40
15 chips = 1 oz (Frito Lay)	1 oz	160	90	56
Corn fritters ✔	1 oz	62	18	29
Enchilada sauce, mild or hot (Del Monte)	1/2 cup	39	1	3
Enchilada, beef ✔	6 oz	317	187	59
cheese ✔	6 oz	320	170	53
chicken ✔	6 oz	240	68	28
Enchiladas, frozen (El Charrito)				
beef	11 oz	560	270	50
cheese	11 oz	470	180	38
chicken	11 oz	440	117	27
Fajita, Beef, frozen (Weight Watcher)	6.75 oz	260	54	21
Green chilies (Old El Paso)	1 oz	7	0	0
Guacamole dip	1 cup	403	297	74
Jalapeno peppers, chopped	1/2 cup	17	tr	tr
Manwich, canned, Mexican (Hunt-Wesson)	1/4 cup	32	0	0
Nachos (Taco Bell)	1 serving	346	167	48
Pintos and Cheese (Taco Bell)	1 serving	190	78	41
Quesadilla ✔	5 oz	739	429	58
Refried beans, plain or spicy	1 cup	248	16	6
vegetarian	1 cup	225	34	15
Salsa Picante, hot or mild (Del Monte)	1/4 cup	15	0	0
Sopaipillas, 3" x 3"	1 piece	141	107	76
Spanish Rice ✔	1/2 cup	217	81	37
Taco (Taco Bell)	1 taco	183	97	53
soft	1 taco	228	106	47
Taco, beef ✔	1 taco	288	153	53
chicken ✔	1 taco	231	90	39

FOOD	AMOUNT	CALORIES		
		TOTAL	FAT	%FAT
Taco chips, 10 chips = 1 oz (Tostitos)	1 oz	140	72	51
Taco salad with salsa (Taco Bell)	1 salad	941	552	59
Taco sauce	1/2 cup	28	2	7
Taco shell, hard	1 shell	48	20	42
Tamale pie, without meat ✔	1 cup	176	71	40
Tamale				
with beef and sauce ✔	1 tamale	244	98	40
with cheese and sauce ✔	1 tamale	244	93	38
with chicken and sauce, 4" tube ✔	1 tamale	164	65	40
with sauce, without meat, 4" tube ✔	1 tamale	139	57	41
(Old El Paso)	2 tamales	232	114	49
Tortilla, soft				
6" diameter				
corn	1 tortilla	63	5	8
flour	1 tortilla	95	18	19
whole wheat	1 tortilla	97	16	16
8" diameter, flour	1 tortilla	127	24	19
Tostada, with beef and refried beans	1 tostada	239	130	54
(Taco Bell)	1 serving	243	100	41

NUTS AND SEEDS

FOOD	AMOUNT	TOTAL	FAT	%FAT
Almonds, whole				
22 = 1 oz	1 oz	153	137	90
5 oz = 1 cup	1 cup	765	684	89
Brazil nuts, whole				
3 = 1 oz	1 oz	173	159	92
5.3 oz = 1 cup	1 cup	916	840	92

FOOD

CALORIES

	AMOUNT	TOTAL	FAT	%FAT
Cashews, 18 = 1 oz	1 oz	161	115	71
5 oz = 1 cup	1 cup	805	575	71
Chestnuts, fresh, 4 large or 6 small	1 oz	58	4	7
Coconut				
fresh, 1 x 1 x 3/8"	1 piece	54	47	87
shredded, 3.4 oz	1 cup	349	303	87
dried, shredded, 2.2 oz	1 cup	344	218	63
Filberts or hazelnuts, whole				
20 = 1 oz	1 oz	183	161	88
4.8 oz = 1 cup	1 cup	878	773	88
Macadamia nuts, whole				
12 = 1 oz	1 oz	206	199	97
4.8 oz = 1 cup	1 cup	988	955	97
Peanut butter, crunchy or smooth	1 Tbsp	95	72	76
	1 cup	1520	1152	76
Peanuts				
chopped	1 Tbsp	52	40	77
dry roasted	1 oz	174	122	70
5 oz = 1 cup	1 cup	868	612	71
roasted in shell, jumbo size	1 nut	11	8	73
Virginia or Spanish				
45 = 1 oz	1 oz	169	129	76
5 oz = 1 cup	1 cup	844	644	76
whole, without shell	1 oz	140	73	52
5.4 oz = 1 cup	1 cup	756	394	52
Pecans, halves				
20 = 1 oz	1 oz	195	182	93
3.8 oz = 1 cup	1 cup	742	693	93
Pine nuts or pinon nuts	1 oz	156	104	67
2.5 oz = 1 cup	1 cup	388	260	67
Pistachio nuts, with shell				
4.4 oz = 1 cup	1 cup	748	607	81
50 = 1 oz	1 oz	170	138	81
Pumpkin or squash seeds				
138 = 1 oz	1 oz	115	87	76
5.4 oz = 1 cup	1 cup	620	472	76

FOOD   CALORIES

	AMOUNT	TOTAL	FAT	%FAT
Sesame seeds	1 Tbsp	48	42	88
Sunflower seeds, shelled	1 Tbsp	51	39	76
400 small seeds = 1 oz	1 oz	158	110	70
5.4 oz = 1 cup	1 cup	853	594	70
Tahini, sesame seed butter	1 tsp	45	27	60
Trail Mix				
Cross Country	1 oz	144	95	66
	1/2 cup	533	351	66
Tropical	1 oz	104	34	33
	1 lb	1644	544	33
	1/2 cup	302	99	33
regular	1 oz	132	73	55
	1 lb	2112	1168	55
	1/2 cup	330	183	55
Walnuts, black, halves				
14 = 1 oz	1 oz	179	156	87
4.4 oz = 1 cup	1 cup	788	668	85
English, halves				
14 = 1 oz	1 oz	185	164	89
3.5 oz = 1 cup	1 cup	648	574	89

ORIENTAL FOODS

	AMOUNT	TOTAL	FAT	%FAT
Almond cookie, Chinese, 2" diameter	1 cookie	153	97	63
Bamboo shoots, fresh	1/2 cup	18	2	11
Barbeque pork, without bone	1 oz	54	32	59
Barbeque spareribs, meat only	1 oz	145	107	74

FOOD	AMOUNT	CALORIES		
		TOTAL	FAT	%FAT
Bean sprouts, mung, raw or cooked	1/2 cup	18	tr	tr
Beef and vegetable stir-fry with rice ✔	1 1/2 cups	513	189	37
Beef teriyaki ✔	4 oz beef	429	315	73
Beef with pea pods, Chinese	1 cup	321	203	63
Cabbage, Chinese, cooked	1/2 cup	12	tr	tr
raw	1/2 cup	6	tr	tr
Chicken teriyaki ✔	1/2 cup	266	160	60
Chicken with almonds, Chinese	1 cup	408	220	54
Chicken with broccoli, Chinese	1 cup	361	225	62
Chicken with cashew nuts, Chinese	1 cup	408	220	54
Chicken with mushrooms, Chinese	1 cup	328	183	56
Chinese beef with tomato ✔	1 cup	265	198	75
Chinese fortune cookies	1 cookie	66	36	55
Chop suey, with meat, canned	1 cup	223	103	46
Chow mein noodles, hard, canned	1 cup	220	108	49
Chow mein				
Chicken, frozen (Stouffer's)	8 oz	140	45	32
chicken, without noodles	1 cup	255	90	35
shrimp, without noodles	1 cup	221	90	4
vegetable, frozen (La Choy)	1 cup	69	3	4
Dim Sum, 4 oz ✔	1 roll	345	189	55
Egg flower soup, Chinese	1 cup	59	27	46
Egg foo yung	1 cup	257	160	62
Egg roll				
chicken, frozen (La Choy)	3 rolls	69	26	38
frozen, restraurant style	3 oz	180	54	30
shrimp, frozen (La Choy)	3 rolls	62	21	34
Fortune cookie, Chinese	1 cookie	66	36	55
Fried rice, with pork				
(Chun King)	1 cup	144	57	40
Chinese ✔	1 cup	312	166	53
Hom Bow				
with chicken, steamed dumpling	1 whole	124	41	33
with pork, steamed dumpling	1 whole	176	70	40
Mandarin Chicken, frozen (Budget Gourmet)	10 oz	290	54	19
Moo goo gai pan ✔	1 cup	566	307	54

FOOD

CALORIES

	AMOUNT	TOTAL	FAT	%FAT
Noodles, chow mein, canned	1 cup	220	108	49
Oriental Beef with vegetables and rice, frozen (Lean Cuisine)	8 5/8 oz	250	63	25
Oriental noodles, Ramen, 3 oz = 1 pkg	1 pkg	390	153	39
Party mix, Oriental	1 oz	150	81	54
Rice cakes	1 cake	35	3	9
Shrimp foo yung	1 cup	288	189	66
Snow or sugar pea pods, fresh	1/2 cup	26	1	4
Soy sauce, regular or lite	1 Tbsp	10	tr	tr
Spicy sour hot soup, Chinese	1 cup	79	35	44
Sweet and sour pork, Chinese	1 cup	344	209	61
Sweet 'n Sour Chicken with Rice, frozen (Budget Gourmet)	10 oz	350	63	18
Tofu, soybean curd	1/2 cup	81	43	53
Water chestnuts, Chinese, raw	4 nuts	20	1	5
Won Ton soup ✔	1 cup	205	31	15
Won Ton, pork, fried	1 piece	59	40	68

P IES

	AMOUNT	TOTAL	FAT	%FAT
Apple cobbler ✔	3/4 cup	505	198	39
Apple pie				
(Burger King)	1 serving	305	108	35
(McDonald's)	1 serving	260	133	51
Apple pie, double crust ✔				
1/6 of 9"	1 piece	403	174	43
1/8 of 9"	1 piece	302	131	43
9", whole	1 pie	2416	1044	43

FOOD

CALORIES

	AMOUNT	TOTAL	FAT	%FAT
Apple pie, snack size (Sara Lee)	1 pie	230	81	35
Apple turnover, 3 oz	1 turnover	255	127	50
Banana cream pie ✔				
1/6 of 9"	1 piece	413	168	41
1/8 of 9"	1 piece	309	126	41
9", whole	1 pie	2478	1008	41
Black bottom pie ✔				
1/6 of 9"	1 piece	576	252	44
1/8 of 9"	1 piece	432	189	44
9", whole	1 pie	3456	1512	44
Blackberry pie, double crust ✔				
1/6 of 9"	1 piece	383	156	41
1/8 of 9"	1 piece	287	117	41
9", whole	1 pie	2296	936	41
Blueberry pie, double crust ✔				
1/6 of 9"	1 piece	381	153	40
1/8 of 9"	1 piece	286	114	40
9", whole	1 pie	2287	919	40
Boston cream pie ✔				
1/6 of 8"	1 piece	415	114	27
1/8 of 8"	1 piece	311	86	28
8", whole	1 pie	2490	686	28
Cherry pie, double crust ✔				
1/6 of 9"	1 piece	411	160	39
1/8 of 9"	1 piece	308	120	39
9", whole	1 pie	2466	961	39
Chocolate cream pie ✔				
1/6 of 9"	1 piece	360	156	43
1/8 of 9"	1 piece	270	117	43
9", whole	1 pie	2160	936	43
Chocolate meringue pie ✔				
1/6 of 9"	1 piece	382	164	43
1/8 of 9"	1 piece	287	123	43
9", whole	1 pie	2293	983	43
Cobbler, apple ✔	3/4 cup	505	198	39

FOOD

CALORIES

	AMOUNT	TOTAL	FAT	%FAT
Coconut cream pie ✔				
1/6 of 9"	1 piece	697	324	46
1/8 of 9"	1 piece	523	243	46
9", whole	1 pie	4184	1944	46
Custard pie ✔				
1/6 of 9"	1 piece	401	196	49
1/8 of 9"	1 piece	301	147	49
9", whole	1 pie	2408	1174	49
Graham cracker crust, 8"	1 crust	1125	646	57
Lemon cream pie ✔				
1/6 of 9"	1 piece	327	144	44
1/8 of 9"	1 piece	245	108	44
9", whole	1 pie	1960	864	44
Lemon meringue pie ✔				
1/6 of 9"	1 piece	357	129	36
1/8 of 9"	1 piece	268	96	36
9", whole	1 pie	2142	771	36
Mincemeat pie, double crust ✔				
1/6 of 9"	1 piece	672	352	52
1/8 of 9"	1 piece	504	264	52
9", whole	1 pie	4032	2112	52
Peach pie, double crust ✔				
1/6 of 9"	1 piece	402	152	38
1/8 of 9"	1 piece	301	113	38
9", whole	1 pie	2410	910	38
Pecan pie, single crust ✔				
1/6 of 9"	1 piece	575	283	49
1/8 of 9"	1 piece	431	212	49
9", whole	1 pie	3449	1700	49
Pecan pie, snack size (Sara Lee)	1 pie	260	117	45
Piecrust, double crust ✔				
1/6 of 9"	1/6 crust	300	176	59
1/8 of 9"	1/8 crust	226	132	58
9", whole	2 crusts	1800	1056	59
Piecrust, mix, double crust, 9"				
10 oz pkg	1 pkg	1485	818	55

FOOD

CALORIES

	AMOUNT	TOTAL	FAT	%FAT
Piecrust, single crust ✔				
1/6 of 9"	1 piece	150	88	59
1/8 of 9"	1 piece	113	66	58
9", whole	1 crust	900	528	59
Pumpkin pie, single crust ✔				
1/6 of 9"	1 piece	320	153	48
1/8 of 9"	1 piece	240	115	48
9", whole	1 pie	1920	920	48
Rhubarb pie, double crust ✔				
1/6 of 9"	1 piece	399	152	38
1/8 of 9"	1 piece	299	113	38
9", whole	1 pie	2391	910	38
Sour cream-raisin pie, single crust ✔				
1/6 of 9"	1 piece	683	270	40
1/8 of 9"	1 piece	513	203	40
9", whole	1 pie	4100	1620	40
Strawberry pie, single crust ✔				
1/6 of 9"	1 piece	245	88	36
1/8 of 9"	1 piece	184	66	36
9", whole	1 pie	1469	527	36
Strawberry-rhubarb pie ✔				
1/6 of 9"	1 piece	576	228	40
1/8 of 9"	1 piece	432	171	40
9", whole	1 pie	3456	1368	40
Sweet potato pie, single crust ✔				
1/6 of 9"	1 piece	323	154	48
1/8 of 9"	1 piece	243	116	48
9", whole	1 pie	1938	925	48

FOOD

CALORIES

	AMOUNT	TOTAL	FAT	%FAT

POULTRY

Chicken franks, 10 = 1 lb	1.6 oz	117	79	68
Chicken gizzards, simmered	1 gizzard	34	7	21
Chicken heart, simmered	1 heart	6	2	33
Chicken liver, simmered	1 oz	44	14	32
Chicken luncheon meat (Land O'Frost)	1 oz	60	36	60
Chicken Nuggets (Kentucky Fried Chicken)	1 piece	46	26	56
Chicken Nuggets, breaded (Swanson)	3 oz	250	144	58
Chicken Patty, breaded (Country Pride)	3 oz	232	135	58
Chicken, boned, canned	1 oz	57	30	53
Chicken, breast, baked				
without skin, 3 oz	1 breast	142	30	21
with skin, 3.5 oz	1 breast	193	68	35
Chicken, breast, batter fried	1 breast	364	167	46
Chicken, light meat				
baked, without skin	1 oz	47	10	21
raw, without skin	1 oz	33	5	15
fried, with skin, without breading	1 oz	67	25	37
cubes, baked, without skin	1/2 cup	116	21	18
Chicken, dark meat				
baked, without skin	1 oz	58	25	43
raw, without skin	1 oz	37	12	32
cubes, baked, without skin	1/2 cup	123	39	32
fried, without skin, without breading	1 oz	75	35	47
Chicken, diced				
dark meat, 1 cup = 4.5 oz	1 cup	261	113	43
white meat, 1 cup = 4.5 oz	1 cup	211	45	21
Chicken, drumstick, baked				
with skin, 1.75 oz	1 piece	112	52	46
without skin, 1.5 oz	1 piece	87	37	43
Chicken, thigh, baked				
without skin, 1.75 oz	1 thigh	109	51	47
with skin, 2 oz	1 thigh	153	86	56

FOOD		CALORIES		
	AMOUNT	TOTAL	FAT	%FAT
Chicken, wing, baked				
without skin, 1/2 oz	1 wing	29	12	41
with skin, 1 oz	1 wing	99	59	60
Chicken, fried ✔	4 oz meat	218	99	45
Chicken, ground, cooked	1 oz	49	30	61
Cornish game hen				
baked without skin	1 oz	40	10	25
raw, with skin	1 whole	400	198	50
Duck, domestic				
raw, without skin	1 oz	38	15	39
roasted, with skin	1 oz	95	72	76
without skin	1 oz	57	29	51
Goose, baked				
with skin	1 oz	86	56	65
without skin	1 oz	67	32	48
Gravy				
chicken or turkey ✔	1/4 cup	128	97	76
chicken, canned	1/4 cup	47	31	66
turkey, dry mix, reconstituted	1/4 cup	22	5	23
Liver pate, chicken	1 Tbsp	69	59	86
Liver, chicken, simmered	1 oz	47	11	23
Pheasant, raw	1 oz	43	13	30
Poultry skin, baked	1 oz	122	91	75
Turkey				
breast, barbecued (Louis Rich)	1 oz	40	9	23
dark meat, roasted, without skin	1 oz	58	21	36
diced, dark meat, 1 cup = 4.5 oz	1 cup	261	95	36
diced, white meat, 1 cup = 4.5 oz	1 cup	225	45	20
ground, raw (Golden Farms)	1 oz	40	18	45
ground, 10% fat, cooked	1 oz	51	21	41
15% fat, cooked	1 oz	60	34	57
hickroy smoked breast (Louis Rich)	1 oz	35	7	20
honey roasted breast (Louis Rich)	1 oz	35	7	20
light meat, roasted, without skin	1 oz	50	10	20
pressed (Land O'Frost)	1 oz	50	27	54
Turkey bologna	1 oz	57	39	68

FOOD		CALORIES		
	AMOUNT	TOTAL	FAT	%FAT
Turkey franks, 8 = 1 lb (Louis Rich)	1 frank	130	90	69
Turkey ham	1 oz	37	13	35
Turkey luncheon meat (Land O'Frost)	1 oz	50	27	54
Turkey pastrami (Louis Rich)	1 oz	35	14	40
Turkey roll, light and dark meat	1 oz	42	18	43
Turkey salami (Louis Rich)	1 oz	55	36	65
Turkey summer sausage (Louis Rich)	1 oz	55	32	58

PUDDINGS AND GELATIN DESSERTS

Bread pudding with raisins ✔	1/2 cup	209	60	29
Custard, baked, with 3.8% milk ✔	1/2 cup	153	66	43
Custard pudding				
with 2% milk (Jell-O)	1/2 cup	153	30	20
with skim milk (Jell-O)	1/2 cup	133	9	7
Flan	1/2 cup	180	79	44
Gelatin				
dry	1 Tbsp	34	tr	tr
sugar free, all flavors (Jell-O)	1/2 cup	8	0	0
with sugar, all flavors (Jell-O)	1/2 cup	80	0	0
Mousse ✔				
chocolate	1/2 cup	246	191	78
strawberry	1/2 cup	248	195	79
Pudding, all flavors				
with 1% milk (Jell-O)	1/2 cup	140	12	9
with 2% milk (Jell-O)	1/2 cup	150	21	14
with skim milk (Jell-O)	1/2 cup	133	0	0
Pudding, bread, with raisins ✔	1/2 cup	209	60	29

FOOD	AMOUNT	CALORIES		
		TOTAL	FAT	%FAT
Pudding, instant mix				
sugar free, with 2% milk	1/2 cup	90	18	20
with 1% milk (Jell-O)	1/2 cup	150	12	8
with 2% milk (Jell-O)	1/2 cup	160	21	13
with 3.8% milk (Jell-O)	1/2 cup	180	36	20
with skim milk (Jell-O)	1/2 cup	143	0	0
Pudding, mix				
with skim milk (D-Zerta)	1/2 cup	70	0	0
with 3.8% milk (Jell-O)	1/2 cup	170	36	21
Pudding, rice				
with 2% milk (Jell-O)	1/2 cup	160	30	19
with raisins ✔	1/2 cup	160	31	19
with skim milk (Jell-O)	1/2 cup	143	9	6
Pudding, tapioca				
with 2% milk (Jell-O)	1/2 cup	160	30	19
with 3.8% milk ✔	1/2 cup	110	35	32
with skim milk (Jell-O)	1/2 cup	133	9	7
Vanilla Pudding ✔	1/2 cup	271	117	43

SALAD BAR

	AMOUNT	TOTAL	FAT	%FAT
Alfalfa sprouts	2 Tbsp	3	tr	tr
Bacon bits	1 Tbsp	38	14	37
Beets, pickled, canned	1/8 cup	20	tr	tr
Broccoli, chopped	1/8 cup	3	tr	tr
Carrots, sliced	1/8 cup	6	tr	tr

FOOD		CALORIES		
	AMOUNT	TOTAL	FAT	%FAT
Cheddar cheese, grated	2 Tbsp	56	42	75
Chickpeas, garbanzo or ceci beans	2 Tbsp	42	5	12
Coleslaw, with mayonnaise dressing	1/2 cup	103	88	85
Cottage cheese, creamed	1/4 cup	59	22	37
Cucumbers, sliced	2 Tbsp	3	tr	tr
Egg, chopped	2 Tbsp	27	17	63
Green pepper, chopped	2 Tbsp	3	tr	tr
Lettuce, chopped	1/4 cup	2	tr	tr
Mushrooms, sliced	1/4 cup	5	tr	tr
Onions, raw, sliced or chopped	2 Tbsp	7	tr	tr
Pocket/pita bread	1 whole	163	7	4
Potato salad, with egg and mayonnaise	1/2 cup	181	92	51
Three bean salad	1/4 cup	77	32	42
Tomato, sliced	3 slices	9	tr	tr

SALAD DRESSINGS

	AMOUNT	TOTAL	FAT	%FAT
Avacado dressing ✔	1 Tbsp	34	27	79
Bleu cheese salad dressing				
reduced calorie	1 Tbsp	11	7	64
regular	1 Tbsp	71	66	93
Buttermilk creamy dressing	1 Tbsp	80	72	90
Buttermilk dressing ✔	1 Tbsp	41	32	78
Caesar salad dressing	1 Tbsp	70	63	90
Catalina salad dressing				
reduced calorie	1 Tbsp	16	0	0
Coleslaw dressing	1 Tbsp	70	54	77
Creamy cucumber dressing	1 Tbsp	70	63	90
reduced calorie	1 Tbsp	25	18	72

FOOD		CALORIES		
	AMOUNT	TOTAL	FAT	%FAT
French salad dressing				
reduced calorie	1 Tbsp	15	9	60
regular	1 Tbsp	65	53	82
Imitation mayonnaise	1 Tbsp	50	45	90
Italian salad dressing				
oil free	1 Tbsp	4	0	0
reduced calorie	1 Tbsp	10	9	90
regular	1 Tbsp	85	80	94
Mayonnaise	1 tsp	33	33	100
	1 Tbsp	100	99	99
Light (Kraft)	1 Tbsp	45	45	100
reduced calorie (Heart Beat)	1 Tbsp	40	36	90
reduced calorie (Weight Watchers)	1 Tbsp	50	45	90
(Saffola)	1 Tbsp	100	99	99
Miracle Whip				
Light (Kraft)	1 Tbsp	45	36	80
regular (Kraft)	1 Tbsp	68	62	91
Oil and vinegar, regular (Kraft)	1 Tbsp	70	63	90
Ranch salad dressing				
reduced calorie	1 Tbsp	40	36	90
regular (Hidden Valley)	1 Tbsp	54	50	93
Russian salad dressing				
reduced calorie	1 Tbsp	27	17	63
regular	1 Tbsp	74	68	92
Sandwich spread, with pickle				
reduced calorie	1 Tbsp	22	16	73
regular	1 Tbsp	76	65	86
Sour cream dressing	1 Tbsp	28	24	86
Tartar sauce, regular	1 Tbsp	75	72	96
Thousand Island salad dressing				
reduced calorie	1 Tbsp	25	18	72
regular	1 Tbsp	80	72	90
Vinaigrette dressing ✔	1 Tbsp	82	81	99

FOOD

CALORIES

	AMOUNT	TOTAL	FAT	%FAT

SALADS

	AMOUNT	TOTAL	FAT	%FAT
Antipasto, raw vegetable ✔	1 cup	355	297	84
Carrot salad				
with nuts, raisins, sour cream	1/2 cup	383	189	49
with raisins and mayonnaise	1/2 cup	141	66	47
Cheddar macaroni salad ✔	1/2 cup	196	117	60
Chef salad				
with 2 Tbsp dressing	2 1/2 cups	480	302	63
without dressing	2 1/2 cups	320	162	51
Chicken salad ✔	1/2 cup	158	72	46
Chicken-stuffed tomato ✔	1 salad	338	225	67
Coleslaw, with mayonnaise-type dressing	1/2 cup	103	88	85
Crab Louis ✔	1 salad	642	495	77
Curried chicken salad ✔	1 cup	582	288	49
Egg salad ✔	1/2 cup	307	249	81
Gelatin salad, with fruit, sweetened	1/2 cup	80	1	1
Greek salad ✔	1 salad	429	342	80
Green salad				
with 1 Tbsp dressing	1 cup	112	73	65
without dressing	1 cup	32	3	9
Ham salad ✔	1/2 cup	287	207	72
Hot five-bean salad ✔	1 cup	293	90	31
Macaroni salad, with mayonnaise ✔	1/2 cup	167	53	32
Pasta salad with vegetables ✔	1/2 cup	100	51	51
Pea salad with cheese ✔	1/2 cup	218	148	68
Potato salad ✔				
hot, German	1/2 cup	139	48	35
with eggs and mayonnaise	1/2 cup	181	92	51

FOOD | CALORIES

	AMOUNT	TOTAL	FAT	%FAT
Raw vegetable antipasto ✔	1 cup	355	297	84
Seven layer salad ✔	1/2 cup	181	137	76
Shrimp salad				
with mayonnaise	1/2 cup	251	205	82
with Miracle Whip salad dressing	1/2 cup	178	118	66
Shrimp-avacado salad ✔	1 2/3 cups	295	162	55
Tabouli	1/2 cup	112	36	32
Taco salad ✔	1/2 cup	141	90	64
Three bean salad ✔	1/2 cup	153	64	42
Tomato aspic salad ✔	1/2 cup	44	1	2
Tossed salad				
with 1 Tbsp dressing	1 cup	112	73	65
without dressing	1 cup	32	3	9
Tuna salad, with egg and mayonnaise ✔	1/2 cup	174	97	56
Tuna-stuffed tomatoes ✔	1 salad	263	162	62
Waldorf salad ✔	1/2 cup	79	56	71

SANDWICHES

	AMOUNT	TOTAL	FAT	%FAT
Bacon, lettuce, tomato sandwich on white	1 sandwich	352	197	56
Bacon Swiss burger (Wendy's)	1 burger	710	396	56
Beef 'n cheddar sandwich (Arby's)	1 sandwich	455	241	53
Big Classic (Wendy's)	1 burger	580	306	53
with cheese (Wendy's)	1 burger	640	360	56
Big Mac hamburger (McDonald's)	1 burger	560	292	52
Big Twin burger (Hardee's)	1 burger	450	225	50
Cheese dog (Dairy Queen)	1 sandwich	330	189	57
Cheeseburger				
(McDonald's)	1 burger	310	124	40
bacon, double (Burger King)	1 burger	510	279	55

FOOD | CALORIES

	AMOUNT	TOTAL	FAT	%FAT
Cheeseburger (continued)				
regular (Burger King)	1 burger	317	135	43
(Wendy's)	1 burger	410	198	48
Chicken club sandwich (Arby's)	1 sandwich	610	297	49
Chicken sandwich	1 sandwich	580	270	47
(Arby's)	1 sandwich	493	225	46
BK Broiler (Burger King)	1 sandwich	379	162	43
(Dairy Queen)	1 sandwich	670	369	55
(Hardee's)	1 sandwich	370	117	32
(McDonald's)	1 sandwich	490	257	53
(Wendy's)	1 sandwich	430	171	40
hot, with 3 Tbsp gravy	1 sandwich	356	138	39
with lettuce on white	1 sandwich	303	126	42
Chili dog (Dairy Queen)	1 sandwich	320	180	56
Club sandwich, chicken (Arby's)	1 sandwich	610	297	49
Corn dog	1 serving	345	202	59
Coney Island ✔	1 sandwich	373	225	60
Corned beef sandwich on rye	1 sandwich	377	182	48
Filet-0-Fish sandwich (McDonald's)	1 sandwich	440	235	53
Fish sandwich				
(Dairy Queen)	1 sandwich	400	153	38
with cheese (Dairy Queen)	1 sandwich	440	189	43
(Hardee's)	1 sandwich	500	216	43
(Skipper's)	1 sandwich	524	297	57
double (Skipper's)	1 sandwich	698	675	94
(Wendy's)	1 sandwich	210	99	47
French dip, 3 oz meat	1 sandwich	461	248	54
Grilled cheese sandwich on white	1 sandwich	430	239	56
Ham 'n cheese sandwich				
(Arby's)	1 sandwich	292	123	42
(Burger King)	1 sandwich	471	207	44
hot (Hardee's)	1 sandwich	330	108	33
Hamburger, double (Dairy Queen)	1 burger	530	252	48
Hamburger, regular				
(Burger King)	1 burger	275	108	39
(McDonald's)	1 burger	260	86	33

FOOD		CALORIES		
	AMOUNT	TOTAL	FAT	%FAT
Hamburger, single				
(Dairy Queen)	1 burger	360	144	40
(Wendy's)	1 burger	350	144	41
Hamburger, triple (Dairy Queen)	1 burger	710	405	57
Hot dog, regular (Dairy Queen)	1 serving	280	144	51
cheese (Dairy Queen)	1 serving	330	189	57
super (Dairy Queen)	1 serving	520	243	47
Mushroom 'n Swiss burger (Hardee's)	1 burger	490	243	50
Patty melt sandwich on rye	1 sandwich	636	383	60
Philly steak sandwich, 3 oz meat	1 sandwich	402	162	40
Quarter Pounder (McDonald's)	1 burger	410	186	45
with cheese (McDonald's)	1 burger	520	263	51
Roast beef sandwich				
super (Arby's)	1 large	501	199	40
regular (Arby's)	1 sandwich	353	133	38
big (Hardee's)	1 sandwich	300	99	33
regular (Hardee's)	1 sandwich	260	81	31
hot, with 3 Tbsp gravy	1 sandwich	429	220	51
Ruben sandwich on rye	1 sandwich	534	267	50
Tuna salad sandwich on white	1 sandwich	320	109	34
Turkey sandwich				
deluxe (Arby's)	1 sandwich	375	149	40
club (Hardee's)	1 sandwich	390	144	37
Whaler (Burger King)	1 sandwich	488	243	50
Whopper (Burger King)	1 burger	628	324	52
with cheese (Burger King)	1 burger	711	387	54

FOOD | CALORIES

	AMOUNT	TOTAL	FAT	%FAT

SOUPS

	AMOUNT	TOTAL	FAT	%FAT
Bean with bacon soup (Campbell's)	1 cup	145	32	22
Bean with pork soup, with water	1 cup	170	54	32
Beef broth				
condensed (Campbell's)	1 cup	46	0	0
reconstituted, with water (Campbell's)	1 cup	23.	0	0
Beef noodle soup	1 cup	65	27	42
Beef-barley soup ✔	1 cup	343	189	55
Black bean soup (Campbell's)	1 cup	110	18	16
Bouillabaisse ✔	1 cup	245	84	34
Bouillon cube, dehydrated	1 cube	5	tr	tr
Chicken and rice soup	1 cup	48	11	23
Chicken consomme or broth	1 cup	22	5	23
condensed	1 cup	44	2	5
Chicken gumbo soup (Campbell's)	1 cup	52	9	17
Chicken soup, hearty (Progresso)	1 cup	118	29	25
Chicken noodle o's (Campbell's)	1 cup	70	18	26
Chicken noodle soup (Campbell's)	1 cup	61	18	30
dry, reconstituted	1 cup	53	11	21
Chicken noodle soup (Progresso)	1 cup	110	29	26
Chicken vegetable-noodle soup ✔	1 cup	295	90	31
Clam chowder				
Manhattan (Campbell's)	1 cup	70	9	13
New England (Campbell's)				
with 3.8% milk	1 cup	157	54	34
with water	1 cup	77	18	23
Consomme	1 cup	29	0	0
Cream of broccoli soup ✔	1 cup	169	99	59
Cream of celery soup (Campbell's)				
with 3.8% milk	1 cup	181	94	52
with skim milk	1 cup	143	54	38
with water	1 cup	86	44	51
Cream of chicken soup				
homemade ✔	1 cup	282	162	57
condensed	1 cup	218	126	58

FOOD

CALORIES

	AMOUNT	TOTAL	FAT	%FAT
Cream of chicken soup (continued)				
with 3.8% milk	1 cup	189	94	50
with skim milk	1 cup	152	54	36
with water	1 cup	109	54	50
dry, reconstituted	1 cup	107	48	45
Cream of mushroom soup, condensed	1 cup	194	108	56
with 3.8% milk	1 cup	178	94	53
with skim milk	1 cup	140	54	39
with water	1 cup	97	54	56
Cream of potato soup				
homemade ✔	1 cup	191	91	48
with water (Campbell's)	1 cup	70	27	39
Egg flower soup, Chinese	1 cup	59	27	46
French onion soup ✔	1 cup	283	108	38
Gazpacho ✔	1 cup	186	108	58
Green pea soup, with water (Campbell's)	1 cup	150	9	6
Ham and bean vegetable soup	1 cup	126	27	21
Lentil Soup				
homemade ✔	1 cup	247	45	18
(Progresso)	1 cup	143	29	20
Manhattan clam chowder ✔	1 cup	276	90	33
Minestrone soup				
homemade ✔	1 cup	79	15	19
(Progresso)	1 cup	134	22	16
with water (Campbell's)	1 cup	71	18	25
New England clam chowder ✔	1 cup	327	126	39
(Progresso)	1 cup	185	94	51
Onion soup	1 cup	35	8	23
dehydrated, 1.5 oz	1 pkg	150	45	30
Oyster stew ✔	1 cup	233	138	59
Ramen oriental noodles, with broth, 3 oz = 1 pkg	1 pkg	390	153	39
Spicy sour hot soup, Chinese	1 cup	79	35	44
Split pea soup				
homemade ✔	1 cup	233	54	23
with water	1 cup	145	27	19

FOOD	AMOUNT	CALORIES		
		TOTAL	FAT	%FAT
Tomato soup				
canned, condensed (Campbell's)	1 cup	180	48	27
with 3.8% milk	1 cup	170	67	39
with skim milk	1 cup	132	18	14
with water	1 cup	90	27	30
cream of, homemade ✔	1 cup	189	99	52
Tomato vegetable noodle soup, with water	1 cup	65	9	14
Tomato vegetable soup, dry, reconstituted	1 cup	56	2	4
Vegetable beef soup, with water (Campbell's)	1 cup	69	9	13
Vegetarian vegetable soup, with water (Campbell's)	1 cup	69	9	13
Won Ton soup ✔	1 cup	205	31	15

SUGARS

FOOD	AMOUNT	TOTAL	FAT	%FAT
Brown sugar, packed	1 tsp	17	0	0
	1 Tbsp	51	0	0
	1/2 cup	410	0	0
Honey	1 Tbsp	65	0	0
Molasses				
dark, blackstrap	1 Tbsp	45	tr	tr
light	1 Tbsp	50	tr	tr
sorghum	1 Tbsp	55	tr	tr
Sugar, granulated	1 tsp	15	0	0
	1 Tbsp	45	0	0
	1/2 cup	360	0	0
6 grams = 1 packet	1 packet	23	0	0
Sugar, maple, 1 3/4 x 1 1/4 x 1/2"	1 oz	99	0	0
Sugar, powdered, sifted	1/2 cup	193	0	0

245

FOOD

CALORIES

	AMOUNT	TOTAL	FAT	%FAT
SYRUPS AND TOPPINGS				
Butterscotch caramel topping (Smucker's)	1 Tbsp	45	tr	tr
Chocolate syrup (Hershey)	1 Tbsp	53	2	4
fudge type	1 Tbsp	62	23	37
thin type	1 Tbsp	46	4	9
Corn syrup, light and dark, (Karo)	1 Tbsp	55	0	0
Maple syrup				
imitation flavor	1 Tbsp	59	0	0
real	1 Tbsp	50	0	0
Marshmallow Creme, topping (Kraft)	1 Tbsp	45	0	0
Pancake syrup				
fruit flavored	1 Tbsp	59	0	0
maple flavored	1 Tbsp	59	0	0
reduced sugar, "lite"	1 Tbsp	30	0	0
Strawberry topping (Smucker's)	1 Tbsp	40	tr	tr

VEGETABLES

	AMOUNT	TOTAL	FAT	%FAT
Acorn squash, baked, 1/2 squash	1/2 cup	65	9	14
Alfalfa sprouts	1/2 cup	12	1	8
Artichoke hearts, frozen	1/2 cup	20	tr	tr
Artichokes with butter sauce ✔	1 average	232	207	89
Artichokes				
Jerusalem, small, 1 1/2" diameter	1 small	17	tr	tr
medium	1 medium	53	2	4

FOOD

CALORIES

	AMOUNT	TOTAL	FAT	%FAT
Asparagus				
canned, cut	1/2 cup	22	3	14
fresh or canned, spears,				
1/2" diameter	4 spears	15	tr	tr
Avocado				
cubed	1/2 cup	125	110	88
mashed	1/2 cup	276	243	88
whole, peeled, 4" diameter	1 average	378	333	88
Baked potato				
plain, large (Wendy's)	1 potato	250	18	7
plain, 5 x 2", medium	1 potato	145	2	1
with cheese, bacon (Wendy's)	1 potato	570	270	47
with sour cream, chives (Wendy's)	1 potato	460	216	47
Bamboo shoots				
canned	1/2 cup	11	tr	tr
fresh	1/2 cup	18	2	11
Bean sprouts, mung, raw or cooked	1/2 cup	18	tr	tr
Beans				
green, cut, fresh cooked,				
canned or frozen	1/2 cup	15	tr	tr
yellow, cut, fresh cooked,				
canned or frozen	1/2 cup	18	tr	tr
Beet greens, cooked, leaves and stems	1/2 cup	13	tr	tr
Beets				
canned, pickled	1/2 cup	81	tr	tr
canned, whole baby	1/2 cup	36	tr	tr
fresh cooked,				
canned, sliced or diced	1/2 cup	30	tr	tr
Broccoli				
raw				
chopped	1/2 cup	12	tr	tr
stalk	1 average	42	tr	tr
fresh cooked or frozen				
chopped	1/2 cup	25	tr	tr
stalk	1 average	40	tr	tr
Broccoli and cheese sauce, frozen	1/2 cup	70	18	26

FOOD

CALORIES

	AMOUNT	TOTAL	FAT	%FAT
Brussels sprouts and butter sauce, frozen	1/2 cup	60	9	15
Brussels sprouts, fresh or frozen, cooked	1/2 cup	28	4	14
Cabbage				
green or red, chopped or shredded	1/2 cup	10	tr	tr
green or red, cooked, drained	1/2 cup	15	tr	tr
Savoy, raw, chopped	1/2 cup	8	tr	tr
Candied squash ✔	1/2 squash	164	36	22
Carrots				
fresh cooked,				
canned, sliced, drained	1/2 cup	23	tr	tr
raw, 7 1/2"	1 carrot	30	tr	tr
raw, grated	1/2 cup	23	tr	tr
Cauliflower				
fresh or frozen, cooked	1/2 cup	15	tr	tr
raw, chopped	1/2 cup	16	tr	tr
with cheese sauce, frozen	5 oz	130	63	48
Celery				
diced	1/2 cup	10	tr	tr
large stalk	1 stalk	5	tr	tr
Chayotte, squash, raw	1 medium	56	2	4
Chilies, green	1 Tbsp	4	0	0
Chinese cabbage				
cooked	1/2 cup	12	tr	tr
raw	1/2 cup	6	tr	tr
Cilantro	10 sprigs	2	tr	tr
Collards, fresh or frozen, cooked	1/2 cup	33	4	12
Corn on the cob,				
fresh or frozen, 5" ear	1 ear	118	11	9
Corn, sweet				
canned or frozen, cooked	1/2 cup	70	4	6
canned, cream style	1/2 cup	105	9	9
in butter sauce, frozen	3.3 oz	90	18	20
Cucumber, raw	1 medium	16	2	13
Dandelion greens	1/2 cup	18	4	22
Eggplant, cooked	1/2 cup	19	2	11

FOOD

CALORIES

	AMOUNT	TOTAL	FAT	%FAT
Endive, small pieces	1 cup	10	tr	tr
French fries				
frozen, oven heated	10 pieces	110	34	31
2.5 oz (Arby's)	1 serving	246	119	48
regular (Burger King)	1 serving	227	117	52
large (Dairy Queen)	1 serving	320	144	45
regular (Dairy Queen)	1 serving	200	90	45
regular (Hardee's)	1 serving	230	99	43
(Kentucky Fried Chicken)	1 serving	244	107	44
large (McDonald"s)	1 serving	400	194	49
regular (McDonald's)	1 serving	320	154	48
small (McDonald's)	1 serving	220	108	49
(Skipper's)	1 sering	383	162	42
3 oz (Wendy's)	1 serving	300	135	45
Gardenburger, vegetable patty	1/4 pound	147	46	31
Garlic clove, raw	1 clove	4	tr	tr
Green beans, cut, fresh cooked, canned or frozen	1/2 cup	15	tr	tr
Green onions, scallions, raw, 3/8" diameter	1 onion	3	tr	tr
Green or red pepper, bell				
chopped	2 Tbsp	3	tr	tr
raw	1 large	22	2	9
Hashbrowns				
frozen, not fried (Ore Ida)	6 oz	130	0	0
homemade ✔	1/2 cup	177	81	46
(McDonald's)	1 serving	130	66	51
Hominy				
cooked	1 cup	146	5	3
raw	1 cup	579	16	3
Japanese style in seasoned sauce, frozen	3.3 oz	90	45	50
Jicama, fresh	1/2 cup	48	tr	tr
Kale, fresh or frozen, cooked	1/2 cup	23	4	17
Kohlrabi, fresh, cooked	1/2 cup	18	tr	tr
Lettuce leaves	1 leaf	tr	tr	tr

FOOD

CALORIES

	AMOUNT	TOTAL	FAT	%FAT
Lettuce				
butterhead, 5" diameter	1 head	25	tr	tr
iceberg, 6" diameter	1 head	70	8	11
pieces	1 cup	5	tr	tr
wedge, 1/4 head	1 wedge	15	tr	tr
romaine, chopped	1 cup	10	2	20
lettuce leaves	1 leaf	tr	tr	tr
Lima beans, canned or frozen	1/2 cup	84	2	2
Mashed potatoes, homemade ✔	1/2 cup	81	20	25
Mixed vegetables, canned	1/2 cup	35	tr	tr
Mushrooms				
canned, drained	1/2 cup	26	5	19
raw, sliced	1/2 cup	10	tr	tr
Mustard greens	1/2 cup	15	4	27
Okra pods, 3 x 5/8"	10 pods	30	tr	tr
Onion				
dehydrated flakes	1 Tbsp	13	tr	tr
fresh, cooked	1/2 cup	30	tr	tr
raw, 2 1/4" diameter	1 onion	38	1	3
chopped	1/2 cup	33	tr	tr
sliced	1/2 cup	23	tr	tr
Onion rings				
french fried (Burger King)	1 serving	274	144	53
french fried, 3 oz = 1 serving	1 serving	285	140	49
homemade ✔	10 rings	352	207	59
Onions with cream sauce, frozen	5 oz	140	90	64
Oriental style, frozen	3.3 oz	30	0	0
Oven browned potatoes ✔	1 cup	211	45	21
Parsley	1 Tbsp	tr	tr	tr
Parsnips, fresh cooked	1/2 cup	50	4	8
Pea pods, sugar or snow peas	1/2 cup	26	1	4
Peas				
crowder, shelled	1/2 cup	50	9	18
green, canned, fresh or frozen,				
cooked	1/2 cup	68	3	4
raw, shelled	1/2 cup	56	2	4

FOOD

CALORIES

	AMOUNT	TOTAL	FAT	%FAT
Peas and carrots, frozen	3.3 oz	60	0	0
Peas with cream sauce, frozen	5 oz	180	99	55
Pepper, bell, green or red	1 large	22	2	9
Peppers, hot, chili (Old El Paso)	1 Tbsp	4	0	0
Potato Buds				
instant, dry flakes	1/3 cup	60	0	0
with fat and milk	1/2 cup	130	54	42
Potatoes, baked, with skin, 5 x 2", medium	1 potato	145	2	1
Potato, boiled, without skin, diced	1/2 cup	51	1	2
Potatoes				
au gratin ✔	1/2 cup	177	90	51
hashbrowned	1/2 cup	177	81	46
mashed, homemade ✔	1/2 cup	81	20	25
instant, with fat and milk	1/2 cup	96	32	33
scalloped, without cheese ✔	1/2 cup	127	45	35
Pumpkin, fresh cooked or canned	1/2 cup	40	4	10
Radishes	4 radishes	5	tr	tr
Rutabaga, fresh cooked, cubed	1/2 cup	35	1	3
Sauerkraut, canned	1/2 cup	20	tr	tr
Scallions, green onions, 3/8" diameter	1 onion	3	tr	tr
Shallot bulb, raw, chopped	1 Tbsp	7	tr	tr
Snow or sugar pea pods, fresh	1/2 cup	26	1	4
Spinach, chopped				
canned, fresh or frozen,				
cooked	1/2 cup	23	4	17
raw	1 cup	15	tr	tr
Sprouts, alfalfa	1/2 cup	12	1	8
Squash				
acorn, baked, 1/2 squash	1/2 cup	65	9	14
candied ✔	1/2 squash	164	36	22
summer, all varieties, cooked	1/2 cup	15	tr	tr
winter, all varieties, cooked	1/2 cup	65	4	6
Sweet potatoes				
boiled or baked, with skin, 5 x 2"	1 potato	170	9	5
candied, 2 x 2 1/2"	1 piece	175	27	15
canned, solid pack	1/2 cup	138	4	3

FOOD

CALORIES

	AMOUNT	TOTAL	FAT	%FAT
Swiss chard, cooked, leaves and stalks	1/2 cup	13	2	15
Tater tots, frozen potato (Ore Ida)	4 oz	213	96	45
Tomatillos	1/2 cup	37	4	11
Tomato juice, canned	8 oz	45	tr	tr
Tomatoes				
canned	1/2 cup	25	tr	tr
raw, 3" diameter				
whole	1 tomato	25	tr	tr
sliced	1 slice	3	tr	tr
Turnip greens, fresh or frozen, cooked	1/2 cup	20	tr	tr
Turnips				
fresh, cooked	1/2 cup	18	tr	tr
raw, diced, 3 1/2 oz = 1 cup	1 cup	40	3	8
Vegetable juice cocktail	8 oz	40	3	8
Vegetable stir-fry, meatless ✔	1 cup	94	45	48
Water chestnuts, Chinese, raw	4 nuts	20	1	5
Watercress, raw	10 sprigs	2	tr	tr
Winter squash, cooked	1/2 cup	65	4	6
Yams, boiled or baked, with skin	1/2 cup	105	2	2
Zucchini squash				
cooked, diced	1/2 cup	13	tr	tr
raw, sliced or diced	1/2 cup	11	tr	tr

FOOD		CALORIES		
	AMOUNT	TOTAL	FAT	%FAT

FOOD		CALORIES		
	AMOUNT	TOTAL	FAT	%FAT

FOOD		CALORIES		
	AMOUNT	TOTAL	FAT	%FAT

FOOD		CALORIES		
	AMOUNT	TOTAL	FAT	%FAT

REFERENCES

Better Homes and Gardens. *New Cook Book.* New York: Better Homes and Gardens Books, 1989.

Brownell, K.D. and J.P. Foreyt, eds. *Handbook of Eating Disorders.* New York: Basic Books, Inc., 1986.

Buying Guide for Fresh Vegetables, Herbs and Nuts. Fullerton CA: Blue Goose, Inc., 1976.

Connor, S.L. and W.E. Connor. *The American Diet.* New York: Fireside/Simon and Schuster, 1986.

DeBakey, M.E. and A.M. Gotta Jr., L.W. Scott, J.P. Foreyt. *The Living Heart Diet.* New York: Raven Press/Simon and Schuster, 1984.

Handbook of Food Preparation. 8th ed. Washington, DC: American Home Economics Association.

Home and Garden Bulletin. Nutritive Value of Foods No. 72. United States Department of Agriculture. Human Nutrition Information Service (1986).

Katch, F., and W.D. McArdle. *Nutrition, Weight Control, and Exercise.* Philadelphia, PA: Lea & Febiger, 1988.

Laveille, G.A., M.E. Zabik, and K.J. Morgan. *Nutrients in Foods.* Cambridge, MA: The Nutrition Guild, 1983.

Pennington, J.A.T. *Bowes and Church's Food Values of Portions Commonly Used.* 15th ed. Philadelphia, PA: J.B. Lippincott Company, 1989.

Stevens, V.J., J. Rossner, M. Greenlick, et al. "Freedom from Fat: A Contemporary Multi-component Weight Loss Program for the General Population of Obese Adults." *Journal of the American Dietetic Association* (1989), 89:1254.

Streit, K.J., N.H. Stevens, V.J. Stevens, J. Rossner. "Food Records: A Predictor and Modifier of Weight Change in a Long-term Weight Loss Program." *Journal of the American Dietetic Association,* 1991. (in press)

"The I Can, 101 Cards of Personal Affirmation." Bellevue, WA: G.B.E. Publisher, Inc., 1985.

United States Department of Agriculture. Composition of Foods. Agriculture Handbook No. 8. Washington, DC: Government Printing Office, sec. 1–17. rev. 1976–1989.

United States Department of Agriculture. Nutritive Value of American Foods in Common Units. Agriculture Handbook No. 456. Washing, DC: Government Printing Office, November 1975.

United States Department of Health and Human Services. National Cholesterol Education Program. Eating to Lower Your High Blood Cholesterol. HHS Pub. No. (NIH)89-2920, 1989.

United States Department of Health and Human Services. The Surgeon General's Report on Nutrition and Health. DHHS (PHS) Publication No. 88-50210. Washington, DC: Government Printing Office, 1988.

Note: Nutrient information for products cited in *Health Counts* were obtained from the manufacturer. Brand names, products, and commercial manufactures are mentioned in this publication solely to provide specific information on the fat and calories in the food items. This mention is not an endorsement by Kaiser Permanente.